MARTIAL ART BASICS

ju-jitsu

MARTIAL ART BASICS

ju-jitsu

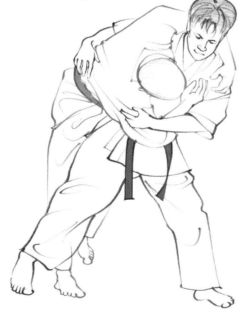

KEVIN PELL
Black belt 8th Dan

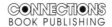

CONNECTIONS
BOOK PUBLISHING

I would like to dedicate this publication to my wife Teresa, my daughter Victoria, my sister Stephanie, my parents, my soul mate, Uke and constant inspiration Ruth Rogers, my very special student and Uchi Deshi Andy Herbert, my best man, business partner and most senior Yudansha Mark Hayden-Smith, and all of my students both past and present, especially my personal and incredible Yudansha and Sempai, Trevor Steward, Andy Tierney, Mark Thomas, Sheila Eglen, Martin Fricker, Lou Panteli and my childhood friend and training partner Brendan King, who, although I lost contact with him many years ago, remains the inspiration behind all that Ishin Ryu Ju-Jitsu has become.

PLEASE NOTE:
The author, packager and publisher cannot accept any responsibility for injury resulting from the practice of any of the principles and techniques set out in this book. A good level of health and fitness is essential in order to practise Ju-Jitsu; if you are in any doubt about your physical condition and ability, please consult a medical professional before attempting these techniques. The author strongly recommends that Ju-Jitsu practice be performed under the supervision of a qualified instructor wherever possible.

A CONNECTIONS EDITION
This edition published in Great Britain in 2011 by
Connections Book Publishing Limited
St Chad's House, 148 King's Cross Road
London WC1X 9DH
www.connections-publishing.com

British Library Cataloguing-in-Publication data available on request.

ISBN 978-1-85906-332-3

1   3   5   7   9   10   8   6   4   2

The text and illustrations in *Martial Art Basics: Ju-Jitsu* were previously published in card deck form in 2005 by Connections Book Publishing (UK), Barnes & Noble Books (US) and Gary Allen (Aus), and first published in book form in 2008 by Grange Books (UK).

Phototypeset in Zurich using QuarkXPress on Apple Macintosh

Printed in China

CONTENTS

INTRODUCTION

Why Ju-Jitsu?

Ju-Jitsu is a highly effective method of self-defence that has a great deal to offer anyone of any age and at any level of ability. It relies on skill and speed rather than strength, so is ideal for men, women and children alike.

People are drawn to Ju-Jitsu for a variety of reasons. For example:

- As a practical method of self-defence
- To develop and maintain a high level of physical stamina, fitness and flexibility
- To improve self-discipline and control
- To increase and focus powers of concentration.

Its core as a practical, no-nonsense art of self-defence is why Ju-Jitsu is currently taking the martial arts world by storm, and now has millions of followers worldwide. The supremacy of Ju-Jitsu techniques has been proven time and time again by its total dominance of the highly publicized ultimate-fight challenges, no-rules and ring-rules competitions – cross-discipline matches where the best martial artists from across the world come to test their skills against each other. No proponent of any other martial art discipline has yet managed to better Ju-Jitsu's techniques. The immense popularity of these events has brought Ju-Jitsu into the lives of millions of people across the world, reinforcing its reputation as a martial art second to none.

This book is the perfect way to supplement your Ju-Jitsu training, whether you are taking up this martial art for the first time or are already an experienced Ju-Jitsu practitioner. Everything from basic breakfalls through to defence against an armed attacker is clearly presented step by step, with concise instructions alongside 'top tips' to help you get the best results from your training. This book can be used any time and anywhere, and will become an invaluable training aid to your study of the fascinating art of Ju-Jitsu.

Origins and history

The origins of Ju-Jitsu can be traced as far back as 712 CE in the ancient chronicles of Japan, and it was widely practised by the Samurai warriors. The noble Samurai followed a strict code of discipline known as *Bushido* – the 'way of the warrior'. This code upheld the very desirable qualities of loyalty, sense of duty, obedience, honor and respect, and it governed their daily lives as well as serving to reinforce their tenacious and resolute fighting spirit in battle.

The classical art of Ju-Jitsu is still alive and well today, perpetuated by a small number of enthusiastic practitioners who wish to keep alive the Samurai spirit and traditional values of the deadly fighting techniques of Ju-Jitsu. Not for them competition born out of the sporting arena – their only goal is the continuation of the mental, spiritual and physical purity of their chosen art.

The Ju-Jitsu practised by the Samurai focused primarily on annihilating the enemy, which subsequently led to the development of many dangerous and fatal techniques that are, understandably, of great interest to modern-day special forces and specialized security agencies. Modern Ju-Jitsu practised as a study of self-defence, although being a highly effective and practical hands-on system, concentrates on defeating an opponent using minimal force together with specially developed arrest and restraint techniques.

Philosophy and spirit

Ju-Jitsu is literally translated as the 'science of softness', even though most of the techniques are extremely dynamic in their delivery and appear anything but soft. This lies behind its central philosophy, which is to overcome an opponent by any and all means with *minimal* force – hence 'softness'. With the emphasis on the practical, Ju-Jitsu relies on a no-nonsense approach to self-defence that teaches practitioners to neutralize an attack and administer a counter-strike – distracting the opponent before taking him or her to the floor with a throw or trip. True to the indomitable fighting spirit, the attacker may then be immobilized using a wide range of arm, shoulder or wrist locks, or with holds or submission techniques such as strangles, chokes and arm locks.

Benefits of Ju-Jitsu

The benefits of the various physical and mental disciplines Ju-Jitsu necessitates are far-reaching, and you will soon notice their influence in other areas of your life. For example:

- **Fitness and flexibility** You will feel the difference as you go about your daily activities – even if it's something as simple as not getting out of breath when you run for a bus or climb a flight of stairs.
- **Confidence and well-being** Within a relatively short period of time your confidence and feeling of general well-being should increase due to the very nature of your Ju-Jitsu training, as you will be working with a number of different partners – both male and female – and engaging in bouts of ground grappling.
- **Practical self-defence skills** Ju-Jitsu quickly teaches you that less is more: for a technique to be effective, it must be both quick and simple.
- **Assertiveness and awareness** These valuable qualities are developed and honed through your training. Within our Ishin Ryu school of Ju-Jitsu we work on the three key letters SAS: **S**peed, **A**ggression, **S**urprise.
- **Stress reduction** Experience has taught me over many years of training that no matter how bad a day you have had, it will never seem as bad after a good training session.
- **Comradeship** Membership to any good Ju-Jitsu club will inevitably bring about a new and tightly knit circle of friends who not only share a common interest but believe in the same ideals and values. A good maxim to remember is 'train hard – play hard'.
- **Self-discipline and a positive attitude** Turning up for training after a hard day's work isn't always easy. However, by regularly making the effort to get to your Ju-Jitsu club, you will find that you become more focused and self-disciplined and also more likely to succeed – not only in the *dojo* (practice hall) but in your day-to-day life too.

Inside the dojo
What to expect

Most Ju-Jitsu classes begin with a formal 'bowing-in' ceremony which, in some schools, may include a couple of minutes of meditation in preparation for the mental as well as physical demands of the class. This will be followed by stretching and a light cardio warm-up, which should include breakfalls. This involves the students performing forward rolls and dropping into left and right breakfalls, which not only forms a crucial part of Ju-Jitsu training but also improves flexibility, confidence and cardiovascular fitness. After this, the instructor will normally gather the students round for technical tuition in a number of self-defence techniques, before the class breaks away into smaller groups according to grade and experience, so that students can study their belt syllabus in preparation for future gradings.

Towards the end of the lesson, the students will engage in a light warm-down – vital to prevent the build-up of lactic acid in the muscles and joints – before the class is concluded with the 'bowing-off' ceremony.

Dojo etiquette

Within the martial arts generally, and certainly within Ju-Jitsu, students are expected to adhere to a strict and formal code of etiquette. This begins from the minute you enter the dojo until you leave, and these principles should also be carried through into your daily life. Dojo etiquette covers a vast and varied range of subjects, including bowing in and out of the dojo – both to your instructor and to senior grades – and understanding the significance of the opening and closing ceremonies within the dojo as well as the rules and observations regarding dress code, cleanliness and presentation of your *dogi* (training uniform). Personal hygiene also plays an important role within Ju-Jitsu, due to the fact that students practise in close proximity with a partner. Practitioners of Ju-Jitsu must ensure that their nails are clean and short, any jewellery is removed and their hair is tied back if necessary.

Students are expected to behave with courtesy and respect at all times, and to listen diligently to the advice and guidance of their instructor.

Clothing and equipment

Ju-Jitsu practitioners usually wear a white wrap-over style heavyweight kimono commonly known as a *dogi* or *gi*. The gi is tied around the middle with a red belt (or belt colour according to grade). It is important to make sure that the suit fits comfortably for reasons of safety and practicality. Thereafter, it becomes equally important to keep your gi clean, presentable and in a good state of repair, and proudly displaying the club's badge or insignia. Groin guards should also be worn (by women as well as men) to aid in preventing serious injury to the groin region. In addition, students should be encouraged to wear *zoris* (traditional-style flip-flops) to and from the edge of the mat, to prevent the contamination of the matted area.

Within your study of Ju-Jitsu, as you progress you can expect to cover a wide and varied range of weapon techniques, both classical and modern, from traditional weapons as used by the Samurai to close-range knife- and pistol-disarm techniques, in response to weapons that one could encounter anywhere in the uncertain world we live in.

Grading

Official gradings are held to test the seniority, experience and knowledge of Ju-Jitsu students. Their achievements are recognized and rewarded through a progressive series of coloured belts, originally devised by the founder of modern-day Judo, Jigoro Kano.

Although the grading syllabus may differ from one school to another, our Ishin Ryu Ju-Jitsu system utilizes the most common *Kyu* grade (below black belt) structure of red belt signifying an upgraded novice, followed by – in

Warming up

It is essential to warm up before training sessions, to avoid potential damage to muscles, tendons and joints by going in 'cold'. I have included a few warm-up exercises here to get you started, covering the arms, shoulders, wrists and legs; there are, of course, many more variations on these drills, but these will give you a good all-round idea of the preparatory measures you need to take.

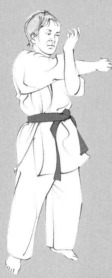

Arm stretch ▶

Hold your right arm out straight, and take it across your upper chest, towards the left. Placing your left forearm on the back of your right upper arm, stretch your arm across your body and hold in this position for a count of 10 seconds. Repeat on the other arm.

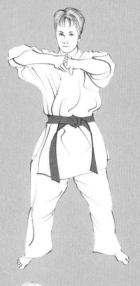

Wrist stretch ▶

Bend your right elbow and hold your arm up in front of you, with your forearm horizontal and your right wrist twisted so that the palm faces outwards. Use your left hand to pull the right wrist in towards your chest, by pulling on the back of the hand. Hold for 10 seconds, then repeat on the other wrist.

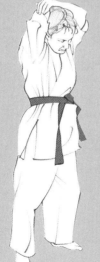

Shoulder stretch ▶

Bend your right arm and stretch it back across your right shoulder to the rear, behind your head, using your left hand on your right elbow for leverage to complete the stretching movement. Hold for a count of 10 seconds, and then repeat on the other shoulder.

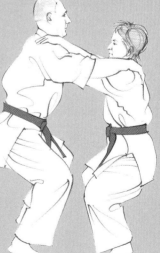

Leg squats ▶

For this exercise you will need to work together with another student. Place your hands on each other's shoulders and, in unison, perform full squats from the standing to the seated position, for up to 40 repetitions.

order – white, yellow, orange, green, blue, purple and brown belts. Following the Kyu grade coloured belts, the student would then sit a *Shodan-Ho* examination, which is a probationary black-belt level (black belt with non-teaching status). This they would hold for a minimum of two years before sitting the coveted black-belt grading, whereupon the successful candidate would be awarded a solid black belt with a single 'first Dan' bar denoting their rank as a Shodan (black belt first Dan). Following on from the student's black belt is the provision for advancement through what is commonly known as the Dan grade system (black belt second Dan, third Dan, and so on).

As with all skills in life, the more practice, dedicated study and continuity you give to your training, the quicker you will progress through your training syllabus and ultimately achieve the coveted black belt, which for many, myself included, signifies the very beginning of understanding the art of Ju-Jitsu.

About this book

Consult the book as and when you need to, to complement your training in class. Carry it around with you as reference for revision purposes, for whenever an opportunity to practise arises, or for when you are uncertain about an element of a technique. Please do not feel that you have to work through the book in any specific order. You will soon learn which aspects of your technique need to be worked on at any given time, so select techniques as appropriate to your training regime. Always read the top tips provided, as they will help you to master the technique. Regular training and constant repetition of your drills is the key to your success.

Advanced Ju-Jitsu

Having mastered the techniques in this book it will be time for you to move on to the next level and, if you haven't done so already, find yourself a reputable club. Ultimately, your success lies in regular training and establishing a realistic and workable training regime. Even if you are only able to train once a week, make sure that you give that session 110 per cent of your effort. Once you have joined a club you will be able to move forward at a good pace. Remember to constantly push yourself mentally and physically – and just when you think you have had enough, push yourself even further.

The major advantage of training in a Ju-Jitsu club is that you have access to a variety of training partners. A common mistake is to train with the same partner continuously. There are no guarantees that in a real-life confrontation your attacker will be your height, your age or your weight, or that you will be attacked by someone of the same sex. When it comes to training, variety is truly the spice of life.

Other important factors to consider if you are going to take your Ju-Jitsu to an advanced level are maintaining a good diet, getting plenty of rest and, of course, constantly striving towards a higher level of physical fitness. Remember that if push comes to shove, you must always be 'fit to fight'.

Practical matters
Finding a club

In my 38 years' martial arts experience, I have found that the number one key to success is finding the right club for you. This is not always as easy as you might think, as sadly the martial arts world has more than its fair share of charlatans ever ready to relieve you of your hard-earned cash and provide you with dubious qualifications. From my experience, the best advice that I am able to offer is 'look around'. Don't just join up at the local club because it happens to be the closest to where you live. Once you have located a prospective club, attend two or three times as a spectator, and have a chat with the students. More often than not, our intuition will guide us in the right direction. Ask yourself a few simple questions. Does the instructor look confident in what he is teaching? Does he seem approachable? Are his students smart and disciplined? Do his students appear to be comfortable and happy with the class? Are his students respectful towards him? Remember that it is sometimes very easy to confuse fear with respect!

Ask the instructor a little about himself. Any instructor worth his salt will have no objection to being questioned in this way and will, in fact, probably open up and speak with passion on his chosen arts, his students and his club. Next comes the question of cost. Don't feel embarrassed to discuss this with the club instructor. You will need to know the cost of your training fees, how much your annual membership will be (and whether it includes insurance cover – more about this below), the cost of training equipment, and what is expected of you in terms of your commitment to the club. It is also a good idea to enquire as to whether the club belongs to a national or international governing body, and who regulates the gradings, and so on.

Insurance

OK – here comes the big one: martial arts insurance! I am fully aware that there are countless instructors around the world teaching martial arts out of local rented premises, and who may escape the eye of the local authorities in terms of insurance. Remember your life is in their hands, and if things go wrong it could be you that has to foot the bill. Always insist on seeing the instructor's professional indemnity insurance as well as his first-aid and coaching qualifications. Ensure that you and all the other students within the club have member-to-member insurance cover, and that you are issued with the appropriate documents and licence.

BREAKFALLS

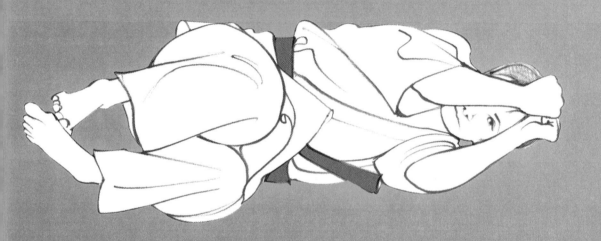

Side breakfall

Before commencing training in any martial art that involves throws and take-downs, it's imperative that the student be taken through some very simple exercises on breaking the initial fall – commonly known within the throwing arts as breakfalls. We'll look at the side breakfall first, which simulates landing on the floor from a throwing technique.

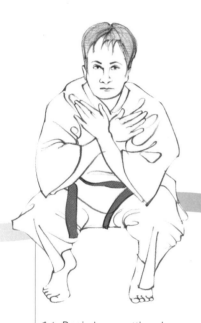

1▲ Begin by squatting down with your backside over your heels, slightly raised on your toes and with your hands crossed over your chest, palms facing towards you.

2▼ Raising up slightly from the crouching position, throw your left leg across your body to the right-hand side, while lifting your left arm above your head in preparation to fall to your left-hand side.

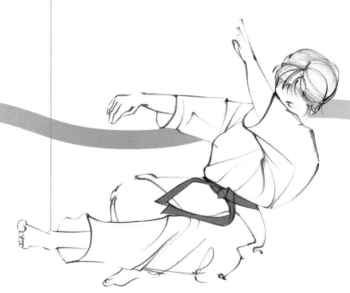

3► As you fall, slap your left hand (palm down) onto the floor in a rapid and assertive manner. It's vital that the arm strikes the floor at right angles to the body just a split second before the body makes contact with the floor.

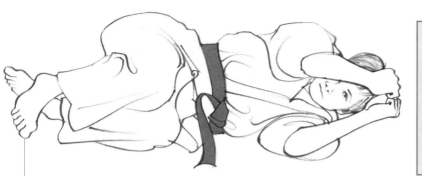

4▲ Having landed in the side breakfall position, immediately clench your fingers to form fists and bring your forearms up in a defensive covering position in front of your face, while your legs cross over to guard against a strike to the groin.

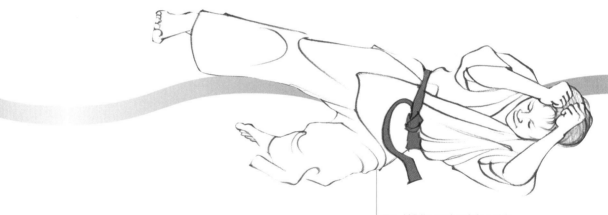

5▲ While maintaining this defensive cover-up stance, draw your right knee up to your chest in preparation to deliver a devastating side stamp kick to your would-be assailant's kneecap, thus incapacitating them.

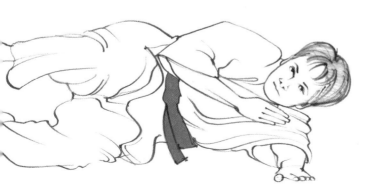

Front breakfall

The front breakfall is commonly used if you are pushed forwards with force, enabling you to land relatively safely by spreading the impact over the length of the arms.

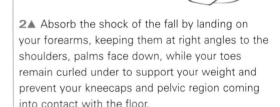

2▲ Absorb the shock of the fall by landing on your forearms, keeping them at right angles to the shoulders, palms face down, while your toes remain curled under to support your weight and prevent your kneecaps and pelvic region coming into contact with the floor.

3▼ Spin rapidly onto your left-hand side, assuming the defensive cover-up posture as used in the side breakfall.

1▲ Standing with your feet together and your hands by your sides, lunge forwards in a dive to the floor.

4▶ The right leg is then once again used to deliver a powerful stamp kick to the attacker's knee or groin region. (NOTE: this position is favoured by right-handed people, as the right leg is generally more powerful. If you find it more comfortable, you can spin onto your right-hand side in step 3, and deliver the final kick with your left leg.)

Rear breakfall

The rear breakfall is useful if you are tripped backwards. As with the front breakfall, you are able to spread the impact over the length of the arms.

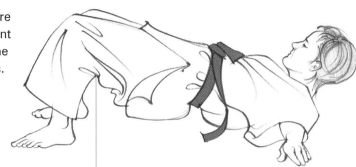

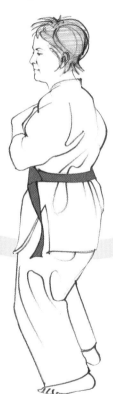

1◄ Standing with your feet shoulder width apart and your arms crossed over your chest, palms facing towards you, lower your backside slightly to the floor and lean back in preparation to fall into the rear breakfall position.

2▲ Having allowed yourself to fall backwards, drive your arms out simultaneously in a crucifix action, striking the floor (palms down) just before your shoulders make contact. Slightly raise your pelvis to prevent your lower back coming into contact with the floor, and make sure your chin is tucked in to prevent your head being driven into the floor when you land.

3▼ Again, bring your arms up, but this time to the side of the temples, with your fingers firmly closed to protect the sides of your head against a follow-up attack. At the same time, draw your right (or left) knee up to your chest in preparation to deliver a front stamp kick to the would-be attacker.

TOP TIP
When falling forwards, make sure you keep your knees, pelvis and chest off the floor by slightly raising your backside (similar to a press-up position on your elbows), thus preventing serious damage to your face and kneecaps.

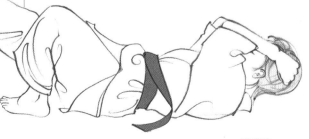

STANCES

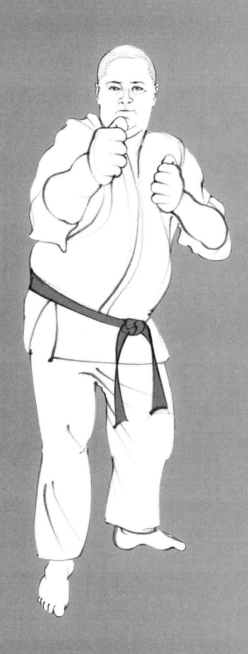

Passive defensive stance

The passive defensive stance is best suited to any situation in which you are confronted with a verbal assault or an attempt to grab at your clothing, or even – in extreme cases – a threat with a close-range weapon. The objective is to lull your attacker into a false sense of security, thus putting him off guard for when you initiate your counter technique.

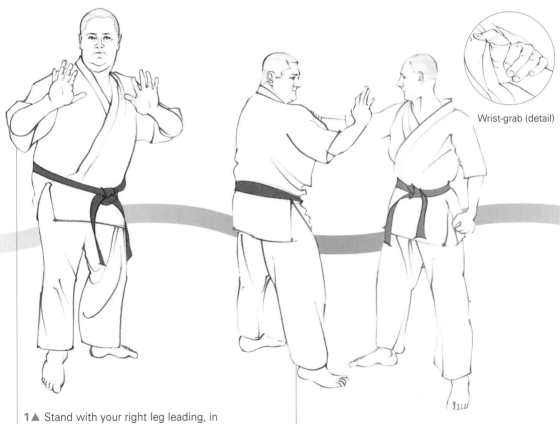

Wrist-grab (detail)

1▲ Stand with your right leg leading, in a 75/25 weight-distribution stance, with the greater proportion of weight on the back leg. Bring your open hands up in front of you in a protective and placatory gesture, with your body leaning slightly backwards, as if cowering away from a potential attack.

2▲ The attacker reaches forwards to grab at your jacket. Immediately bring your left hand up to secure his wrist by wrapping your fingers over the top and pressing on the inside of the wrist (see inset detail). At the same time, step slightly back on the left leg, thus pulling the attacker slightly towards you.

TOP TIP
This stance is invaluable in so many situations, so make sure you use it to your advantage. If your attacker believes that you are of no real threat to him, your counter technique will be all the more effective.

3▼ Drive your right hand forward into the attacker's face using a palm-heel strike, rising slightly upwards to the attacker's nose, so driving his head to the rear and putting him off balance.

4◄ Before the attacker has a chance to react, grab his right shoulder and deliver a front snap kick to the groin region using the instep of your foot.

5▼ Having delivered the kick, you can then drag the attacker forwards off balance, onto the floor.

Guard stance

The guard stance works on the principle of an even weight distribution, ensuring that you are ready to respond to any kind of attack, with the arms extended to create a perimeter defence against the would-be attacker.

TOP TIP
Make sure you have transferred sufficient weight onto the rear leg in step 2 so as to enable the front leg to deliver the kick without major upper-body movement giving the game away.

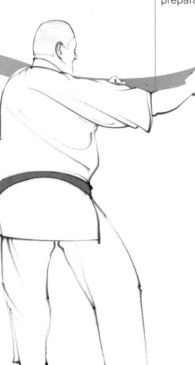

2▼ The attacker attempts to throw a roundhouse punch with his right fist. As he does this, shift your weight onto your rear leg in preparation for your counter attack.

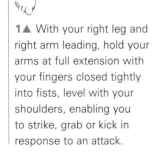

1▲ With your right leg and right arm leading, hold your arms at full extension with your fingers closed tightly into fists, level with your shoulders, enabling you to strike, grab or kick in response to an attack.

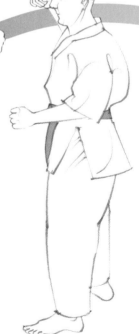

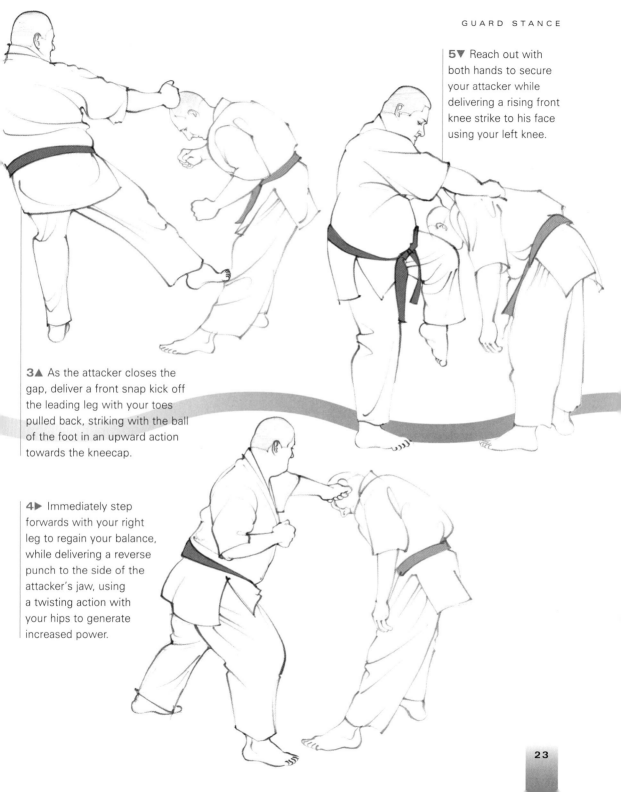

5▼ Reach out with both hands to secure your attacker while delivering a rising front knee strike to his face using your left knee.

3▲ As the attacker closes the gap, deliver a front snap kick off the leading leg with your toes pulled back, striking with the ball of the foot in an upward action towards the kneecap.

4▶ Immediately step forwards with your right leg to regain your balance, while delivering a reverse punch to the side of the attacker's jaw, using a twisting action with your hips to generate increased power.

DEFENCE AGAINST GRABS AND HOLDS

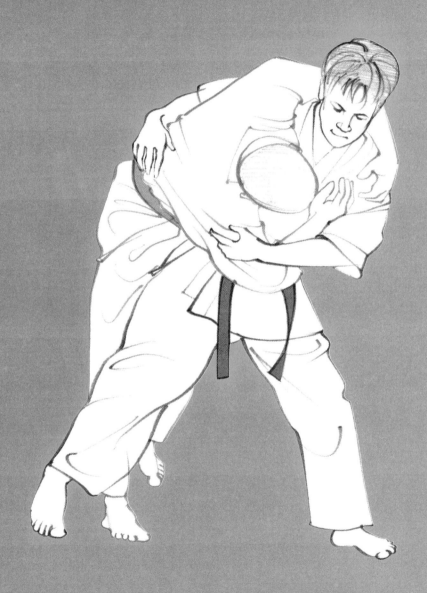

Single-lapel grab

This defence is particularly effective when grabbed by a single grip to the upper body as a threat or an attempt to pull or push you off balance.

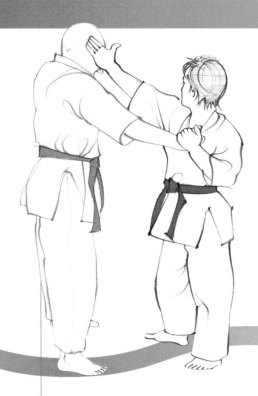

1▼ The attacker reaches out to grab your upper jacket. As he does so, step back on your left foot to assume the passive defensive stance in preparation for your counter-attack.

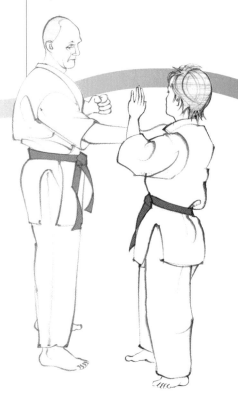

2▲ Stepping further back with your left leg, secure the attacker's wrist with your left hand while delivering a strike to his eyes using a flicking action with the backs of the fingers of your right hand.

> **TOP TIP**
> When taking the attacker to the floor, the elbow and wrist must be maintained on the same level in order for the lock to work to its full effect – which is why it is commonly known as the 'spirit-level lock'.

3▼ Now pull your right hand back to grab the attacker's wrist, freeing up your left hand to grip his elbow.

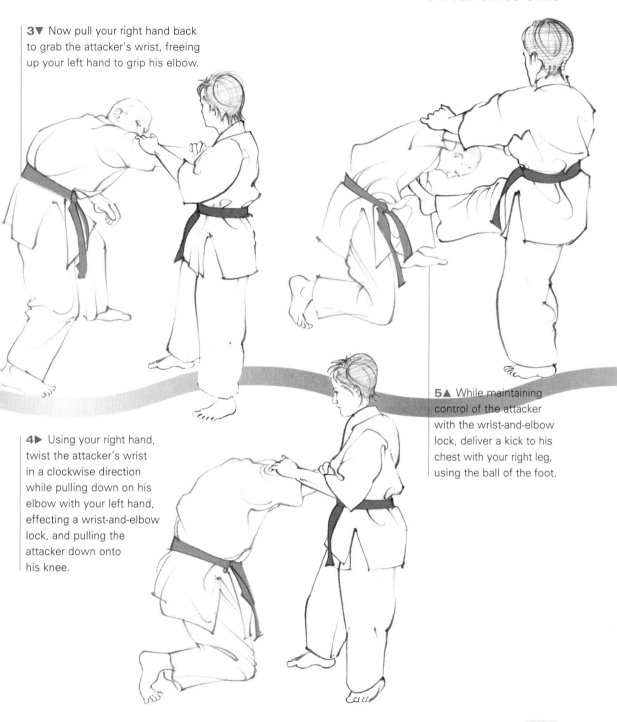

5▲ While maintaining control of the attacker with the wrist-and-elbow lock, deliver a kick to his chest with your right leg, using the ball of the foot.

4▶ Using your right hand, twist the attacker's wrist in a clockwise direction while pulling down on his elbow with your left hand, effecting a wrist-and-elbow lock, and pulling the attacker down onto his knee.

Double-lapel grab

This defence is made against an attacker who secures your clothing with both hands, again in an attempt to pull or push you in a threatening manner.

1▼ The attacker reaches forwards with both hands to grab the top of your clothing, in an attempt to use his head to strike you in the face. As he grabs you, step back slightly with your left leg and raise your open hands into the passive defensive stance.

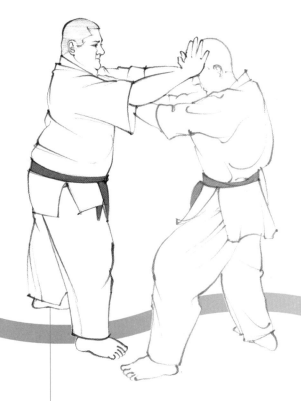

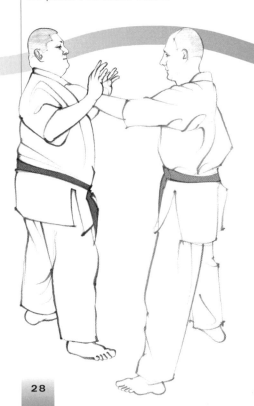

2▲ As the attacker tightens his grip and pulls his head back in preparation to strike you, drive both your open hands forward into his eyes, using a double palm-heel strike.

TOP TIP
The tighter you pull your upper body into the attacker's stomach/chest region in step 3, the easier it will be to lift his legs from under him.

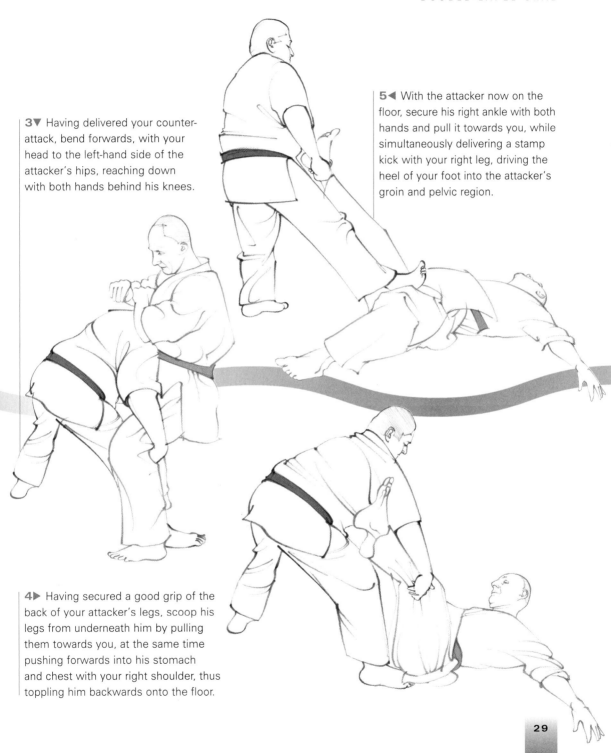

5◄ With the attacker now on the floor, secure his right ankle with both hands and pull it towards you, while simultaneously delivering a stamp kick with your right leg, driving the heel of your foot into the attacker's groin and pelvic region.

3▼ Having delivered your counter-attack, bend forwards, with your head to the left-hand side of the attacker's hips, reaching down with both hands behind his knees.

4▶ Having secured a good grip of the back of your attacker's legs, scoop his legs from underneath him by pulling them towards you, at the same time pushing forwards into his stomach and chest with your right shoulder, thus toppling him backwards onto the floor.

Breaking front strangle (1)

This technique is particularly effective against an attacker who grabs you round the throat using both hands, as you are able to take advantage of their balance and posture and their extended grip.

1▼ The attacker reaches out and grabs you round the throat, pressing both hands on the windpipe. As he does this, step back with your left foot into the passive defensive stance.

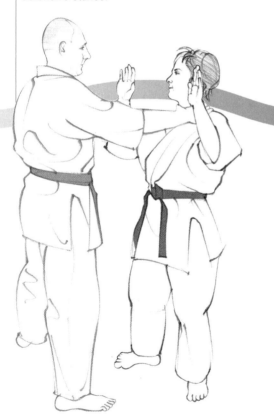

2▲ Immediately step forwards on your left foot, raising your left arm in the air and folding your hand over to simulate the curved handle of an umbrella, which you can then use in a downward action to break the attacker's grip.

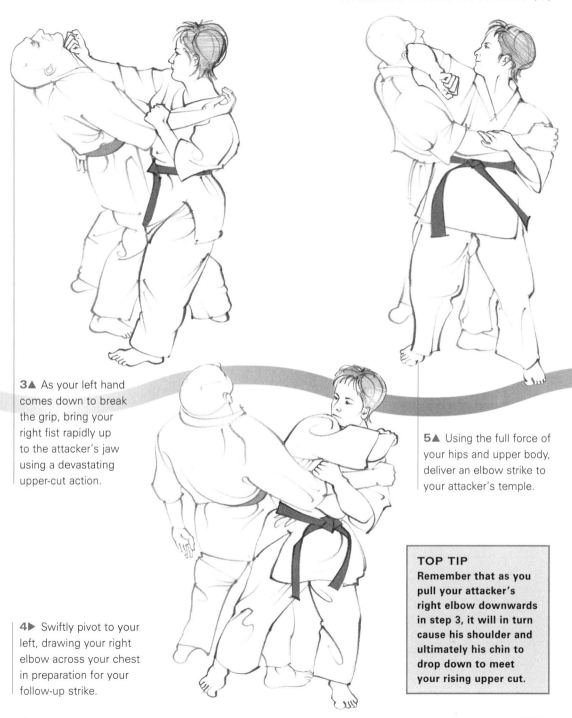

3▲ As your left hand comes down to break the grip, bring your right fist rapidly up to the attacker's jaw using a devastating upper-cut action.

4▶ Swiftly pivot to your left, drawing your right elbow across your chest in preparation for your follow-up strike.

5▲ Using the full force of your hips and upper body, deliver an elbow strike to your attacker's temple.

TOP TIP
Remember that as you pull your attacker's right elbow downwards in step 3, it will in turn cause his shoulder and ultimately his chin to drop down to meet your rising upper cut.

Breaking front strangle (2)

This defence against a double-handed strangle is a particularly effective technique for young children to use, as it relies on body mechanics rather than strength.

1▼ The attacker reaches out and grabs you by the throat using both hands. As she does this, step back on your right leg, clapping your hands together but avoiding interlocking the fingers.

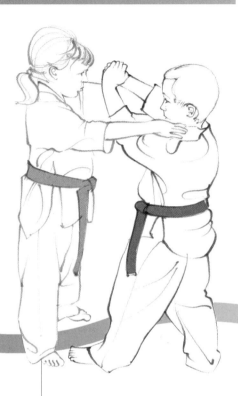

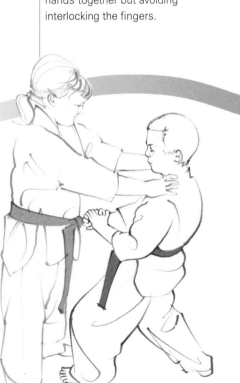

2▲ Using your hips to generate the momentum, drive your arms upwards to form a wedge against the inside of your attacker's elbows.

TOP TIP
Having stepped back after the attacker has grabbed you round the throat it is important to then lower your centre of gravity by bending both knees, to help increase the power of the 'rising wedge' as you drive upwards to break the attacker's grip.

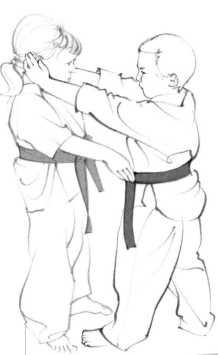

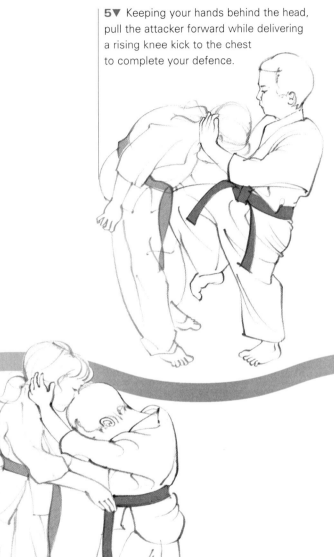

5▼ Keeping your hands behind the head, pull the attacker forward while delivering a rising knee kick to the chest to complete your defence.

3▲ Having broken the grip, reach forwards with your hands to secure your attacker's head in much the same way that you would catch a ball.

4▶ Holding the head securely, drive your head into the attacker's face to put her off guard.

Rear strangle

This technique is ideal for fending off an attack from behind. It shows how best to avoid being held against your will and turn the situation to your advantage.

2▼ Having broken the attacker's grip, step back on your left leg to increase your stability. Cupping your right fist in your left hand, draw on the power of both shoulders to drive your right elbow backwards and upwards into the attacker's sternum.

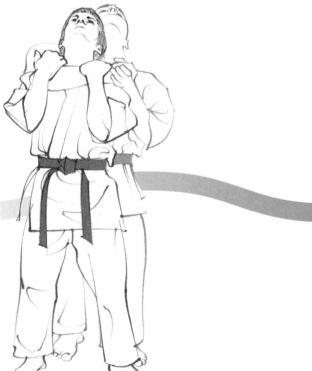

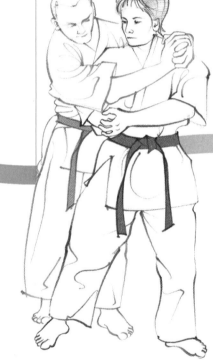

1▲ The attacker grabs you from behind, placing his arm across your throat in order to initiate a choke. Raise your hands and grab his arm to alleviate the pressure on your throat, while driving your head backwards into his face.

> **TOP TIP**
> **Drop your head forwards slightly in step 1 before driving it backwards into the attacker's face, to increase the momentum of the impact.**

3▼ Now side-step to the left, exposing the attacker's groin, and deliver a swift downward-motion chop to this area, striking the attacker firmly between the legs.

4▶ Directly after the strike, while he is still off guard, place your right arm around the attacker's waist and grab his upper sleeve with your left hand, throwing him over your extended right leg.

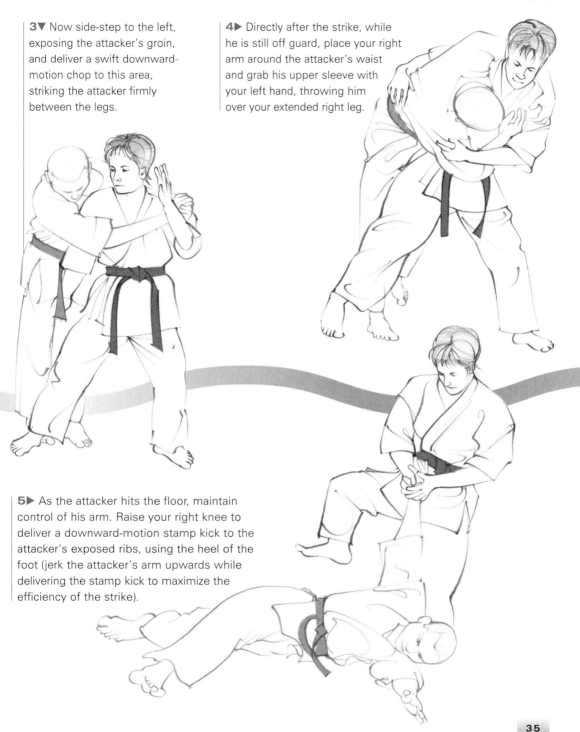

5▶ As the attacker hits the floor, maintain control of his arm. Raise your right knee to deliver a downward-motion stamp kick to the attacker's exposed ribs, using the heel of the foot (jerk the attacker's arm upwards while delivering the stamp kick to maximize the efficiency of the strike).

Rear bear-hug

This technique is ideal for breaking away from an attacker who has secured both your arms in a 'bear-hug' from the rear.

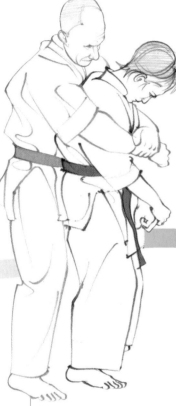

2▼ Having driven the back of your head into the attacker's face, immediately push outwards with your elbows to release the attacker's grip.

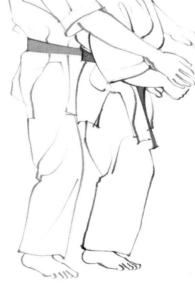

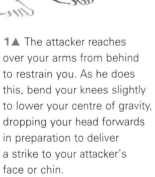

1▲ The attacker reaches over your arms from behind to restrain you. As he does this, bend your knees slightly to lower your centre of gravity, dropping your head forwards in preparation to deliver a strike to your attacker's face or chin.

3▲ Turn sharply to your right, placing your right leg between your attacker's legs and hooking your ankle behind his right leg while gripping the back of the attacker's leg with both hands.

TOP TIP
For your throw to be successful, you must ensure that you trap the attacker's right leg securely with your right foot in step 3, thus enabling you to lift his leg and lean into him to push him off balance.

4▼ Having trapped the attacker's leg, lean into him with your right shoulder, driving him backwards and off balance, landing between his legs as he hits the floor. Immediately counter-strike with a short, sharp blow from your elbow to his floating ribs.

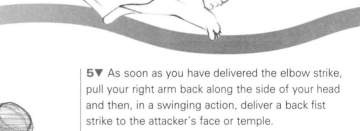

5▼ As soon as you have delivered the elbow strike, pull your right arm back along the side of your head and then, in a swinging action, deliver a back fist strike to the attacker's face or temple.

Side headlock

This technique is particularly effective in dealing with an assailant who has grabbed you in a side headlock in preparation for a take-down or a strike.

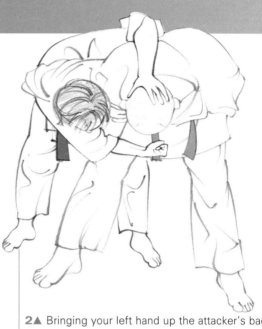

1▼ The attacker steps in and grabs your head in a headlock using his right arm. As he does this, bend your knees to lower your centre of gravity, moving your left leg up close behind his right leg.

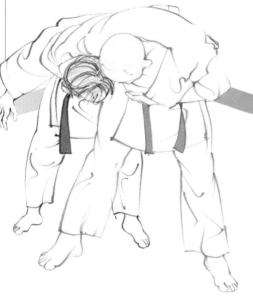

2▲ Bringing your left hand up the attacker's back, strike the back of his head, pushing it forwards, while forming a fist with your right hand and bringing it up to strike him in the face.

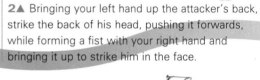

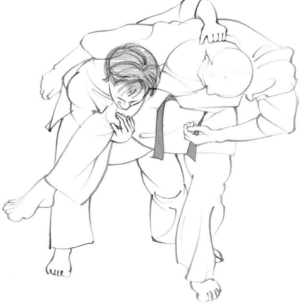

3► Then secure the back of your attacker's collar with your left hand as you step back directly behind him, bringing your right arm between his legs to grab his upper thigh.

4▼ Pushing forwards with your pelvis, lift the attacker's leg and drop him onto the floor.

TOP TIP
Make sure you step in close behind your attacker in step 3, maintaining a firm grip on his upper thigh, and combining a lifting action with a pushing forwards of your hips to maximize the lift.

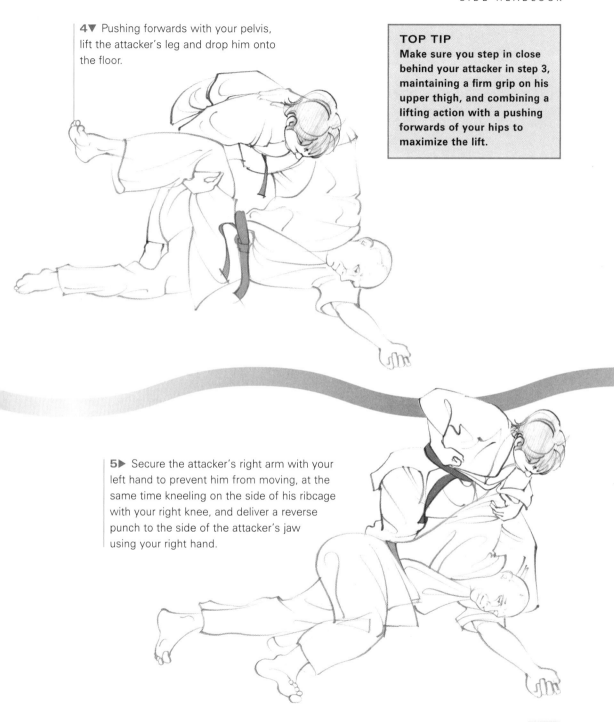

5▶ Secure the attacker's right arm with your left hand to prevent him from moving, at the same time kneeling on the side of his ribcage with your right knee, and deliver a reverse punch to the side of the attacker's jaw using your right hand.

Front headlock

Use this technique when an attacker grabs you from the front, holding you in a front headlock or choke.

3▲ Having delivered the counter strike, wrap your right arm behind the attacker's left leg, at the same time pulling his knees into you as you lean forwards into his stomach.

1▲ The attacker has forced your head down to the side of his body, and has your neck and head firmly locked. Immediately flex your knees to drop your centre of gravity in preparation for your counter move.

2▶ Stepping forwards with your right leg, bring your right arm up between your attacker's legs to strike the groin, while wrapping your left arm around the back of the attacker's right leg.

4▶ While pushing into him with your shoulders, scoop his legs towards you from underneath him, causing him to fall backwards to the floor.

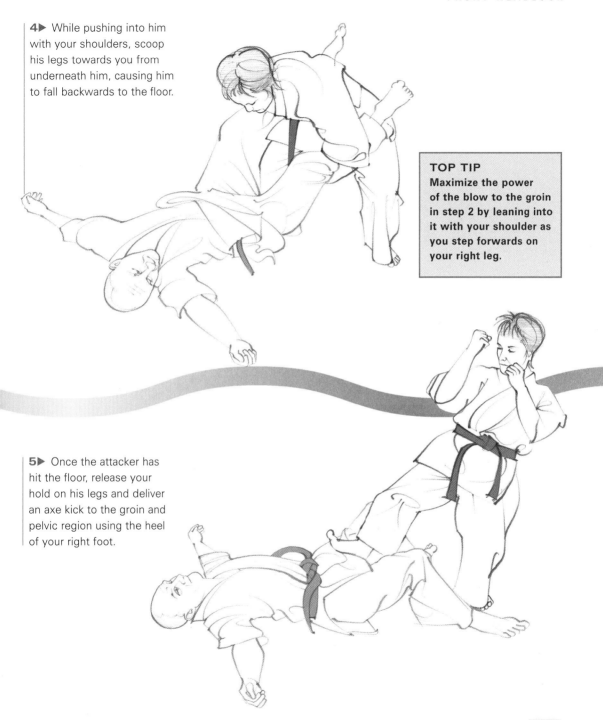

TOP TIP
Maximize the power of the blow to the groin in step 2 by leaning into it with your shoulder as you step forwards on your right leg.

5▶ Once the attacker has hit the floor, release your hold on his legs and deliver an axe kick to the groin and pelvic region using the heel of your right foot.

DEFENCE AGAINST STRIKES

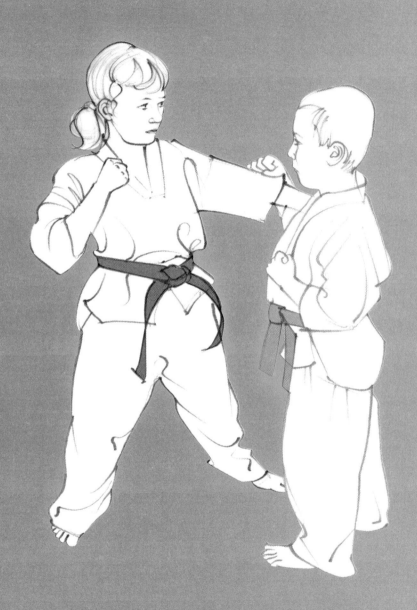

Hip throw with 'JCB' arm lock

This defence should be used against an attacker attempting to make a roundhouse punch to the head.

2▼ Once you have struck the bicep, immediately deliver a strike to your attacker's eyes using the backs of your fingers in a flicking action.

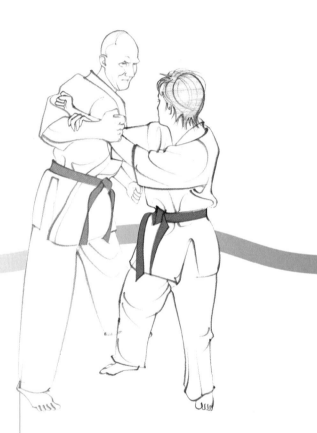

1▲ The attacker attempts to punch you in the head using a roundhouse strike. As the punch comes in, block with your left hand while striking the attacker's bicep with your right hand, using a 'hammer-fist' action.

TOP TIP
The effectiveness of the figure-4 arm lock is maximized by bearing down with both knees onto the attacker's neck and ribs while at the same time lifting his wrist and forearm towards your chest.

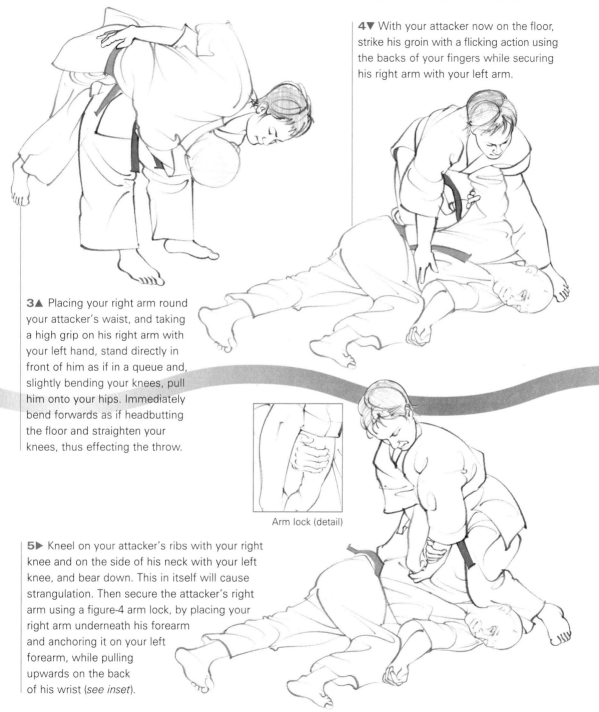

4▼ With your attacker now on the floor, strike his groin with a flicking action using the backs of your fingers while securing his right arm with your left arm.

3▲ Placing your right arm round your attacker's waist, and taking a high grip on his right arm with your left hand, stand directly in front of him as if in a queue and, slightly bending your knees, pull him onto your hips. Immediately bend forwards as if headbutting the floor and straighten your knees, thus effecting the throw.

Arm lock (detail)

5▶ Kneel on your attacker's ribs with your right knee and on the side of his neck with your left knee, and bear down. This in itself will cause strangulation. Then secure the attacker's right arm using a figure-4 arm lock, by placing your right arm underneath his forearm and anchoring it on your left forearm, while pulling upwards on the back of his wrist (*see inset*).

Body drop with shoulder press

This technique is a variation on a defence against a roundhouse punch, this time using a body-drop throw to overpower your attacker.

2▼ Having blocked the punch, pull your right 'hammer fist' back across to the left side of your head and, using a twist of the hips, flick it back to strike the attacker's temple.

1▲ The attacker attempts a roundhouse punch to your head. Block this using your left hand together with a downward hammer blow to the attacker's bicep with your right hand.

3◄ Having delivered the counter strike, step backwards with your left leg so that you are standing in front of your attacker (with your back to him), with your right arm around his waist and your left arm taking a high grip on his right arm. Lunge forwards on your left leg, keeping your right leg straight, and pull your attacker over your extended right leg.

4▶ With your attacker now on the floor, secure his right arm with your left arm, and bring your right knee down onto the back of his right shoulder.

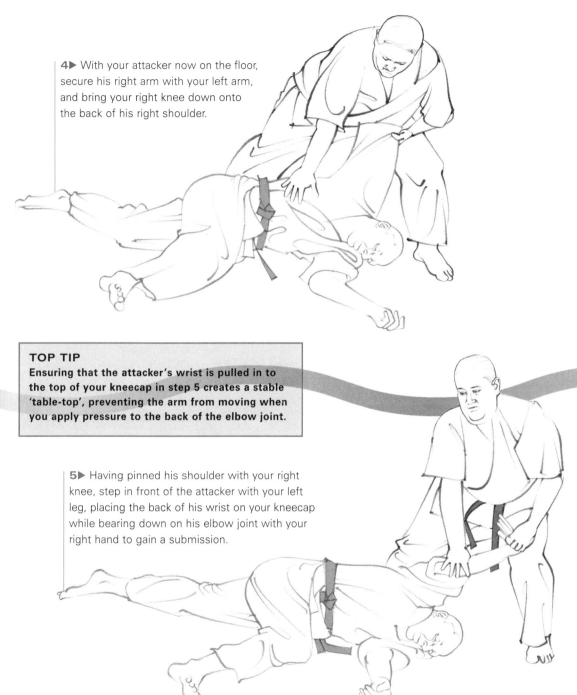

TOP TIP
Ensuring that the attacker's wrist is pulled in to the top of your kneecap in step 5 creates a stable 'table-top', preventing the arm from moving when you apply pressure to the back of the elbow joint.

5▶ Having pinned his shoulder with your right knee, step in front of the attacker with your left leg, placing the back of his wrist on your kneecap while bearing down on his elbow joint with your right hand to gain a submission.

Major outer reap into reclining arm bar

This defence against a punch to the head uses a throwing technique known as major outer reap, due to its sweeping nature. The mechanics of the throw make it particularly effective for children, as the defender does not need to lift the attacker in order to throw them to the floor.

2▼ Having blocked the punch, step forwards on your left foot, at the same time grabbing the attacker's lapel with your right hand and swinging your right leg across and behind him. Sweep his leg away using a pendulum action with your right leg.

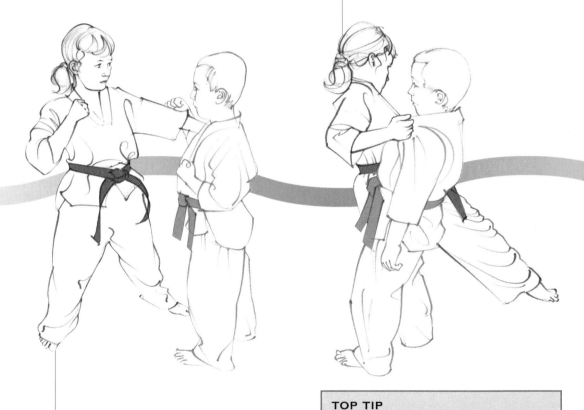

1▲ The attacker attempts to deliver a roundhouse punch to the head. Block the punch using your left arm in a downward chopping action.

> **TOP TIP**
> To maximize the efficiency of the arm bar in step 5, raise your hips off the ground, so as to push your pelvis up, while pulling against the joint in the opposite direction.

3▶ With the attacker now on the floor, stand close to his back and, using both hands, stretch his right arm upwards.

4▶ Now raise your left knee up to enable you to execute a stamp kick to the attacker's jaw with the heel of your left foot. Having delivered the kick, step over the attacker's head with the same leg.

5▼ Maintaining a grip on your attacker's right wrist, drop to your backside and fall backwards, trapping the attacker's arm between your legs, with his elbow joint against your pelvis to effect a straight-arm bar. This allows you either to break the joint (though not in training sessions!) or gain a submission.

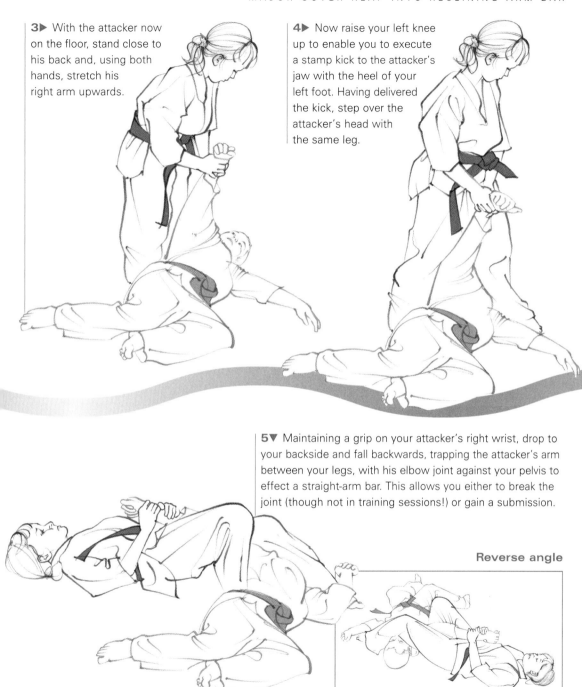

Reverse angle

Sweeping loin with stamp kick

This defence against a strike to the head gives you a series of counter moves with which to overcome your attacker, including a more advanced throw known as the sweeping loin.

2◄ Having blocked the attack, counter strike with your right hand using a 'leopard strike' to the attacker's throat. This involves bending the fingers over and striking with the middle knuckles of the fingers.

3▼ Immediately after delivering the leopard strike, drive your left knee upwards into the attacker's sternum.

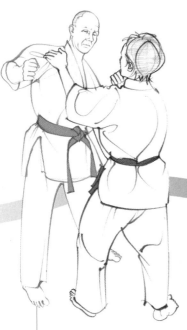

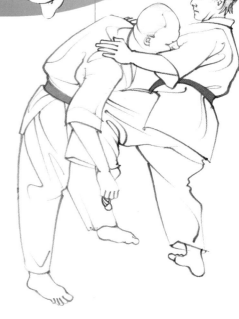

1▲ The attacker attempts to strike you in the head with a punch, which you intercept with a left-handed downward block.

TOP TIP
The success of the sweeping-loin throw is dictated by your ability to maintain the straightness of your leg while bending forwards at the waist and sweeping the attacker's leg away using your right leg.

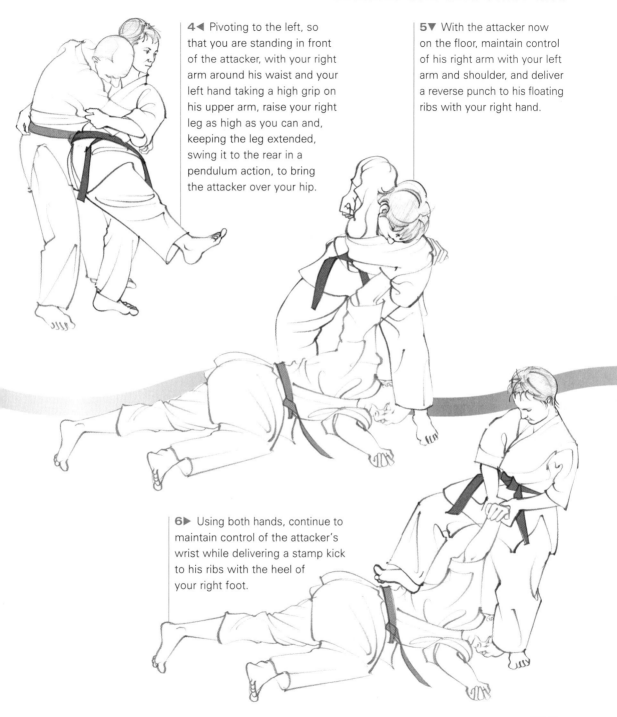

4◄ Pivoting to the left, so that you are standing in front of the attacker, with your right arm around his waist and your left hand taking a high grip on his upper arm, raise your right leg as high as you can and, keeping the leg extended, swing it to the rear in a pendulum action, to bring the attacker over your hip.

5▼ With the attacker now on the floor, maintain control of his right arm with your left arm and shoulder, and deliver a reverse punch to his floating ribs with your right hand.

6► Using both hands, continue to maintain control of the attacker's wrist while delivering a stamp kick to his ribs with the heel of your right foot.

Soccer-kick counter

This technique is an ideal defence against someone attempting to perform a 'soccer kick' (an upward-sweeping kick, as if kicking a ball) aimed at your groin or stomach.

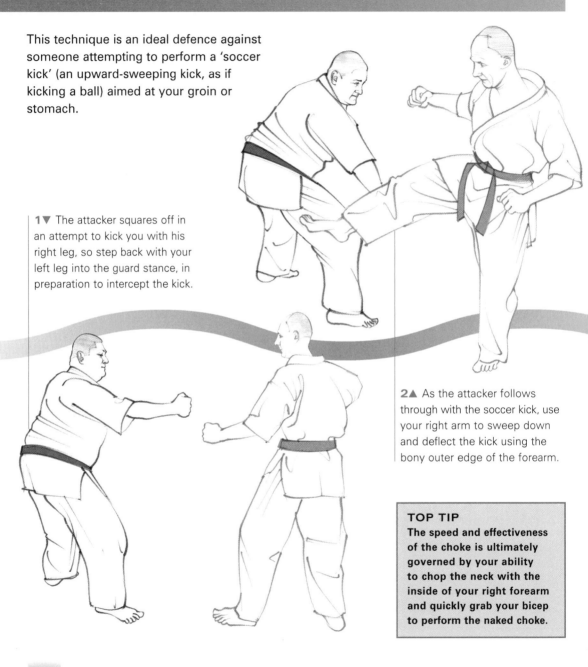

1▼ The attacker squares off in an attempt to kick you with his right leg, so step back with your left leg into the guard stance, in preparation to intercept the kick.

2▲ As the attacker follows through with the soccer kick, use your right arm to sweep down and deflect the kick using the bony outer edge of the forearm.

TOP TIP
The speed and effectiveness of the choke is ultimately governed by your ability to chop the neck with the inside of your right forearm and quickly grab your bicep to perform the naked choke.

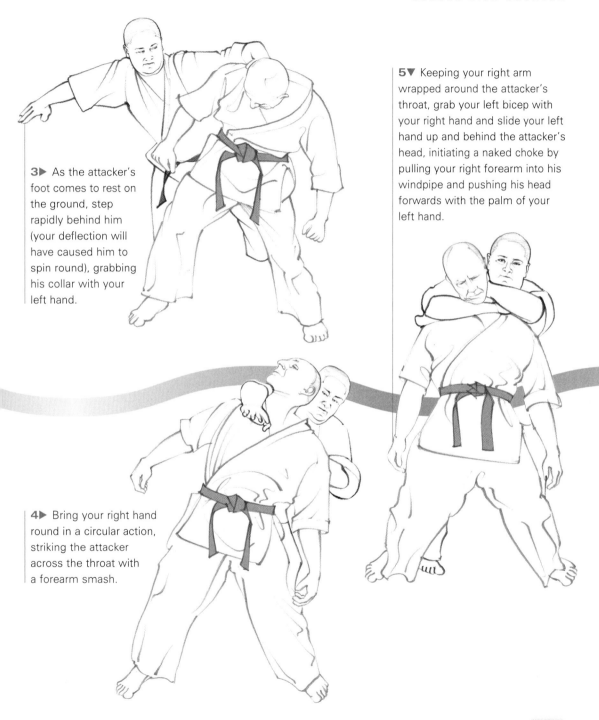

3▶ As the attacker's foot comes to rest on the ground, step rapidly behind him (your deflection will have caused him to spin round), grabbing his collar with your left hand.

5▼ Keeping your right arm wrapped around the attacker's throat, grab your left bicep with your right hand and slide your left hand up and behind the attacker's head, initiating a naked choke by pulling your right forearm into his windpipe and pushing his head forwards with the palm of your left hand.

4▶ Bring your right hand round in a circular action, striking the attacker across the throat with a forearm smash.

Turning-kick counter

This counter-sequence is effective against an aggressor who attempts to deliver a swinging roundhouse kick to your ribs.

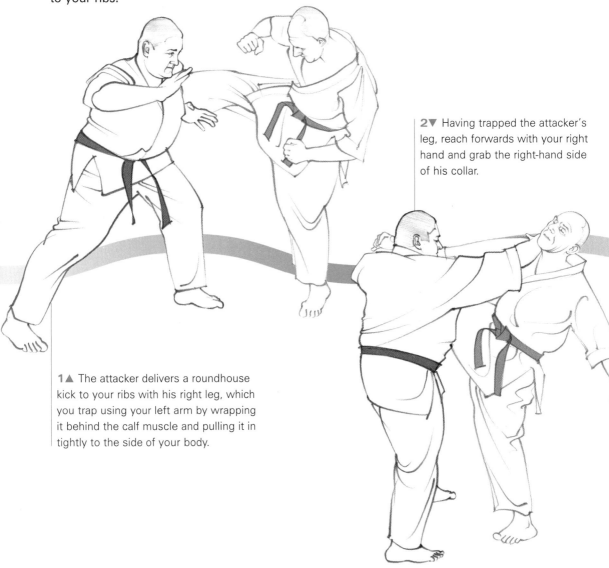

2▼ Having trapped the attacker's leg, reach forwards with your right hand and grab the right-hand side of his collar.

1▲ The attacker delivers a roundhouse kick to your ribs with his right leg, which you trap using your left arm by wrapping it behind the calf muscle and pulling it in tightly to the side of your body.

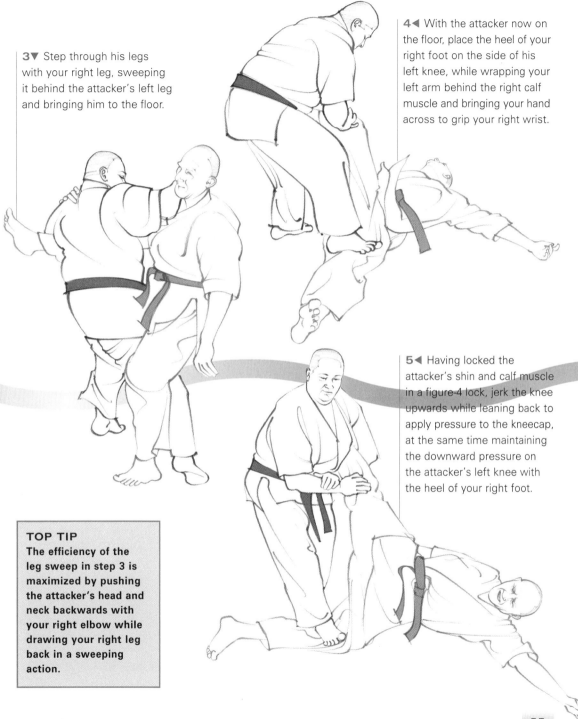

3▼ Step through his legs with your right leg, sweeping it behind the attacker's left leg and bringing him to the floor.

4◄ With the attacker now on the floor, place the heel of your right foot on the side of his left knee, while wrapping your left arm behind the right calf muscle and bringing your hand across to grip your right wrist.

5◄ Having locked the attacker's shin and calf muscle in a figure-4 lock, jerk the knee upwards while leaning back to apply pressure to the kneecap, at the same time maintaining the downward pressure on the attacker's left knee with the heel of your right foot.

TOP TIP
The efficiency of the leg sweep in step 3 is maximized by pushing the attacker's head and neck backwards with your right elbow while drawing your right leg back in a sweeping action.

GROUNDWORK

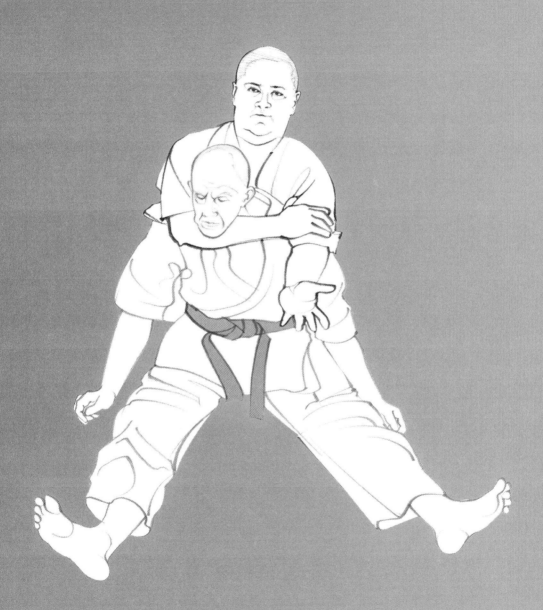

Floor holds

The Ju-Jitsu syllabus includes a vast array of hold-downs. The selection featured here demonstrates some basic hold-down and immobilization techniques which will give you a solid grounding in this area, and which can be applied in a variety of situations.

> **TOP TIP**
> Apply extra pressure to the attacker's head and neck in the upper-four-quarters hold by jamming your hip into the side of the head to push the neck and spine out of alignment, thus weakening the attacker's ability to retaliate.

▶ **SHOULDER HOLD** This can be taken straight from the scarf hold by allowing the attacker's right arm to come free and pushing it across his own neck, then dropping your head behind his arm, so that his arm is sandwiched between the side of your head and his neck. Pull your own head downwards with your right hand to apply further pressure.

▲ **SCARF HOLD** This hold-down is effected by placing your right arm behind the attacker's neck, securing a high grip on his clothing, and wrapping the attacker's right arm around your waist, pulling it in tightly to your body using your arm and elbow. Keep a low centre of gravity and stable base by opening your legs and keeping your head as low as possible to the floor, while bearing down on the attacker's ribcage with the side of your body.

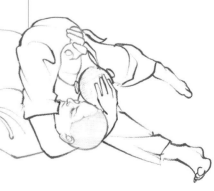

▶ **SHOULDER HOLD FROM THE MOUNT**
Again, a very simple follow-on from the
basic shoulder hold that simply requires
you to sit on top of your attacker
while maintaining the hold and
anchor yourself down by
wrapping your ankles and feet
on the inside of his calf muscles.
Further leverage can be gained on the
choke by pushing back with your legs,
thus lifting your kneecaps off the floor.

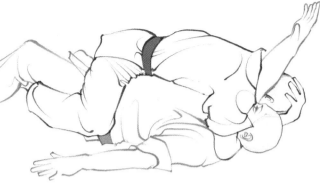

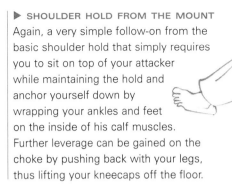

◀ **SIDE FOUR QUARTERS**
This hold-down requires you to
approach your attacker sideways
on by wrapping your left arm
under his head, placing your
palm on the floor, with your right
arm coming between his legs
close to his buttocks, so that
he is unable to use the power
of his leg to break your grip. A
neck lock can be applied to this
immobilization technique by
straightening your left arm,
which will have the effect of
pushing the attacker's head
down towards his knee.

▼ **BROKEN UPPER FOUR QUARTERS** This is ideal when you
find yourself positioned at the upper section of the attacker's
body. Use your right arm to trap the attacker's right arm by
placing it into the top of their collar and holding firmly, while
your left arm pulls back on the attacker's shoulder, preventing
him from being able to use his left arm to any great effect.

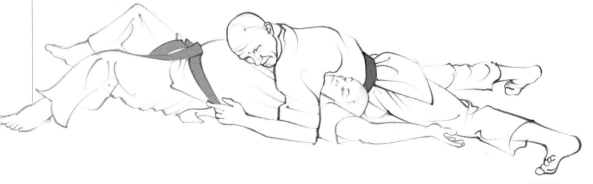

Strangles from the mount

This selection of strangles from the mounted position features techniques that are all very simple to execute, yet extremely effective.

COLLAR AND BAR 1▼ While kneeling down over your attacker, reach across with your right arm and place your fingers deep into the right-hand side of his collar. Then, with your left hand, grab the attacker's left lapel.

▲ **NAKED CHOKE** Sitting astride your attacker, with your knees firmly tucked in to the sides of his chest, place your thumbs on the throat, with one thumb under the adam's apple and one above it. Then, using the tip of the thumb rather than the pad, push both thumbs down simultaneously.

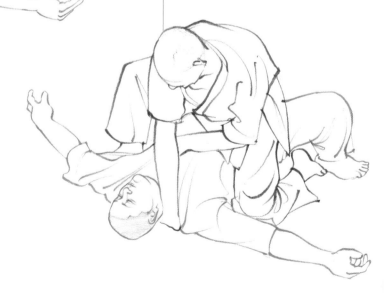

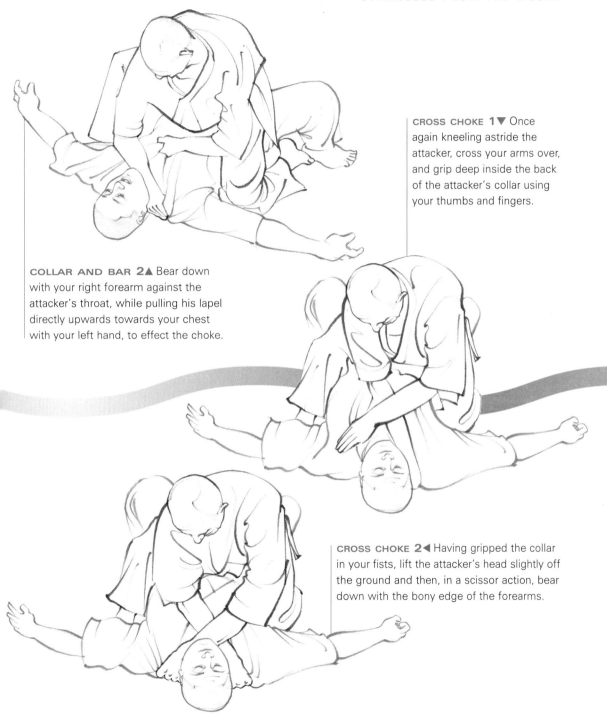

CROSS CHOKE 1▼ Once again kneeling astride the attacker, cross your arms over, and grip deep inside the back of the attacker's collar using your thumbs and fingers.

COLLAR AND BAR 2▲ Bear down with your right forearm against the attacker's throat, while pulling his lapel directly upwards towards your chest with your left hand, to effect the choke.

CROSS CHOKE 2◀ Having gripped the collar in your fists, lift the attacker's head slightly off the ground and then, in a scissor action, bear down with the bony edge of the forearms.

Sprawl

This is a good technique to use when you find that you are able to sit astride your attacker, as it gives you the opportunity to turn him over so that he is face down on the floor, making it ideal to perform a naked choke.

1▲ Sitting astride your attacker with both knees on the floor, pull his left arm across his own chest, and immediately drop onto that arm with your chest in a sprawling action, thus preventing him from being able to move.

2▼ Bring your right hand under the attacker's head and grab hold of his wrist, dragging it towards the side of his head, while placing your left hand on his elbow so that you are able to both push and pull his arm around his head.

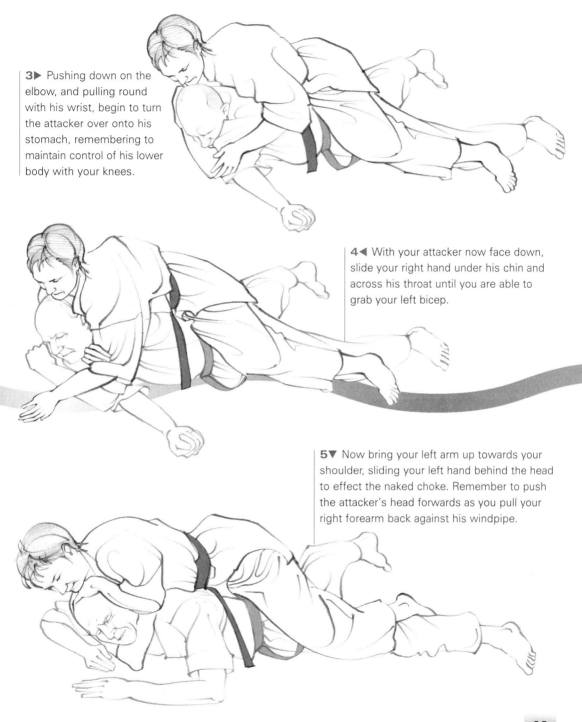

3▶ Pushing down on the elbow, and pulling round with his wrist, begin to turn the attacker over onto his stomach, remembering to maintain control of his lower body with your knees.

4◀ With your attacker now face down, slide your right hand under his chin and across his throat until you are able to grab your left bicep.

5▼ Now bring your left arm up towards your shoulder, sliding your left hand behind the head to effect the naked choke. Remember to push the attacker's head forwards as you pull your right forearm back against his windpipe.

63

Cross-arm lock

This is another highly effective groundwork technique if you find yourself in the dominating upper position, with your attacker on the floor.

2▼ Immediately bend forwards at the waist, putting both your hands on the attacker's chest, and with a sharp pushing-down action, raise your knees off the ground to bring you up into a crouching position.

1▼ The attacker brings his hands up to grab your collar in an attempt to choke you while you are sitting astride him, and thereby regain control of the situation.

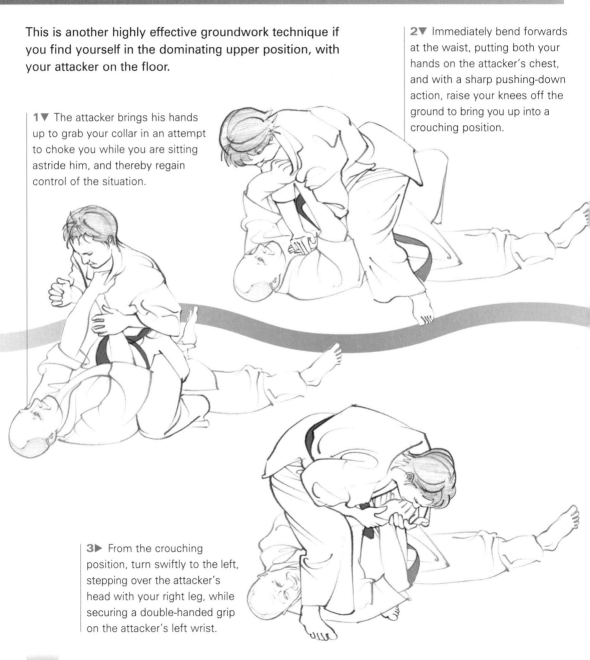

3▶ From the crouching position, turn swiftly to the left, stepping over the attacker's head with your right leg, while securing a double-handed grip on the attacker's left wrist.

4▼ Drop onto your backside and fall back, keeping hold of the attacker's left hand so that his elbow joint is resting on your pelvis, and raise your left leg in preparation to deliver an axe kick to the attacker's sternum using the heel of the foot.

TOP TIP
To maximize the effect of jumping up into the squatting position in step 2, place one hand on top of the other as if administering CPR, and push down fast and hard onto the attacker's sternum.

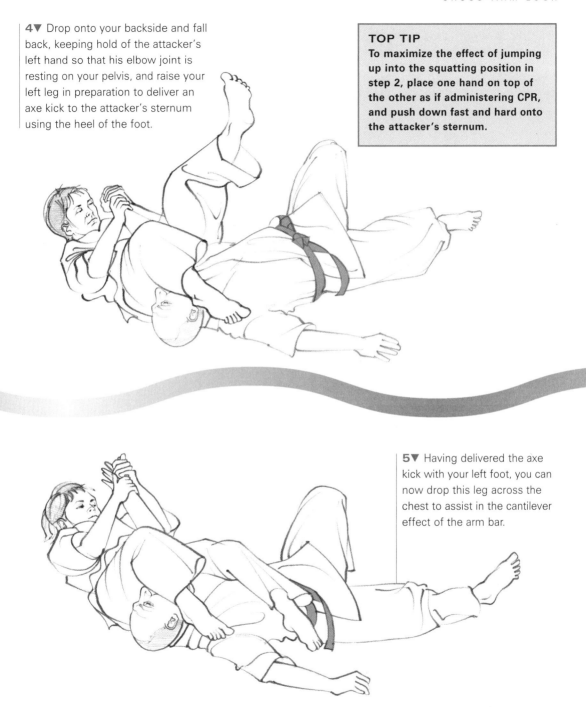

5▼ Having delivered the axe kick with your left foot, you can now drop this leg across the chest to assist in the cantilever effect of the arm bar.

Breaking ground strangle (1)

This sequence of moves demonstrates how best to escape from being held and choked, having been taken to the ground by an attacker, and how to regain control of the situation.

> **TOP TIP**
> To maximize the efficiency of the arm lock in step 3, raise your hips, pushing your pelvis upwards while pulling back on the arm.

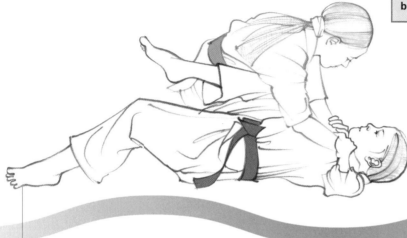

1▲ From a kneeling position, the attacker initiates a strangle with both hands. Place your hands on top of the attacker's, pulling outwards to alleviate the pressure, and raise your right knee, positioning it under the attacker's armpit.

2▼ Ensuring that you maintain control of the attacker by keeping a firm hold on her wrists, swing your left leg upwards and to the rear, bringing it in front of the attacker's face and hooking it behind her head. Then bring your leg down, forcing the attacker backwards onto the floor.

3▶ With both hands now firmly holding the attacker's right wrist, stretch her arm between your legs, positioning the bottom of the elbow joint at the top of your pelvis and thus enforcing a straight-arm bar.

4▶ While still maintaining control of the attacker's wrist and arm, lift your right leg into the air and deliver an axe kick to the attacker's mid-section using the heel of your foot.

5▶ Immediately after delivering the kick, draw your leg back and place your foot on the attacker's side, pushing against her with your foot to roll her away.

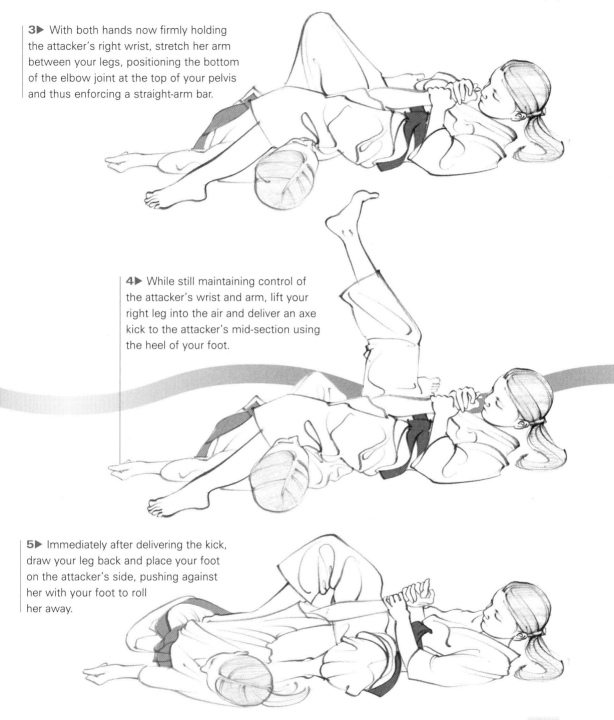

Breaking ground strangle (2)

This is an excellent defence to use against an attacker who is sitting astride you, pinning you to the ground and choking you with both hands.

1▶ The attacker has taken you to the floor and is now sitting astride you, attempting to choke you.

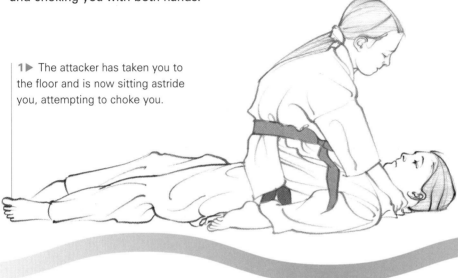

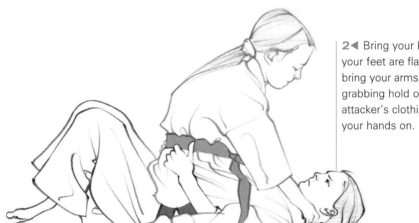

2◀ Bring your knees up so that your feet are flat on the floor, and bring your arms up from your sides, grabbing hold of any parts of your attacker's clothing that you can get your hands on.

3▼ Raising your hips sharply off the ground in an upward thrust while simultaneously pulling as hard as you can on the attacker's clothing, push her upwards and forwards away from you, over your head.

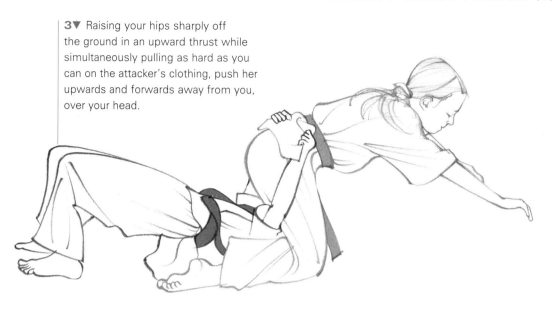

TOP TIP
The effectiveness of the 'throw' in step 3 relies heavily on your ability to thrust up with your hips combined with the determination to pull your attacker over the top of your head, so make sure you give it all you've got.

4▼ With the attacker now face down on the floor, quickly turn onto your left side and, using your right hand, punch up into the groin region.

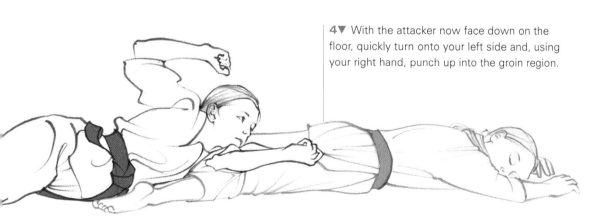

Defence against a kick to the head (1)

This is an ideal technique to use if you find yourself on the floor with an attacker attempting to kick you in the head or face.

2▼ With your right leg, deliver a roundhouse kick to the pit of the stomach, while maintaining your block on the attacker's right leg (either by keeping your forearms on his shin – as here – or by grabbing his trouser leg).

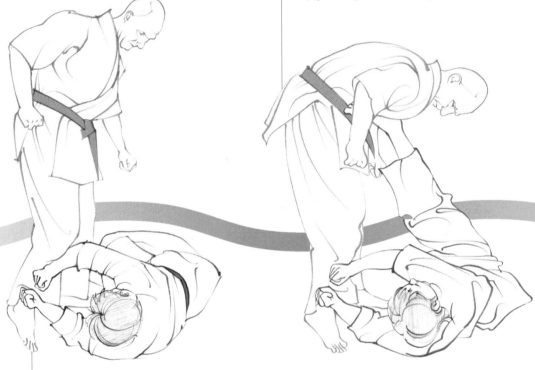

1▲ The attacker has brought you to the ground, and is now attempting to kick you in the face or head. Block the kick by bringing the bony underside of your forearms up in front of your face, so that they make contact with his shin.

TOP TIP
To maximize the effect of the ankle-and-foot lock in step 5, sit bolt upright, pulling the foot into your chest, and pivot sharply to the right, hugging the foot, so that the whole of your upper-body weight is behind the twisting action of the lock.

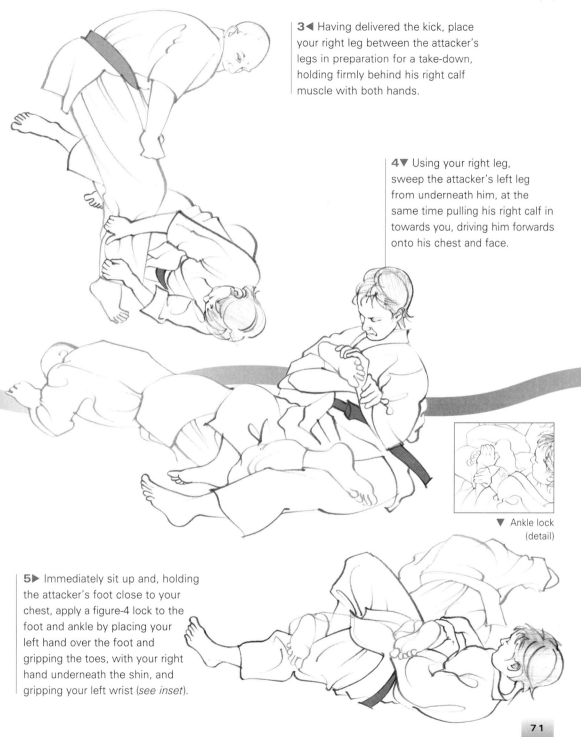

3◄ Having delivered the kick, place your right leg between the attacker's legs in preparation for a take-down, holding firmly behind his right calf muscle with both hands.

4▼ Using your right leg, sweep the attacker's left leg from underneath him, at the same time pulling his right calf in towards you, driving him forwards onto his chest and face.

▼ Ankle lock (detail)

5▶ Immediately sit up and, holding the attacker's foot close to your chest, apply a figure-4 lock to the foot and ankle by placing your left hand over the foot and gripping the toes, with your right hand underneath the shin, and gripping your left wrist (*see inset*).

Defence against a kick to the head (2)

This technique is a variation on a defence against a kick to the head which relies on taking the attacker to the rear rather than pulling him forwards – often easier for those of a smaller build to execute.

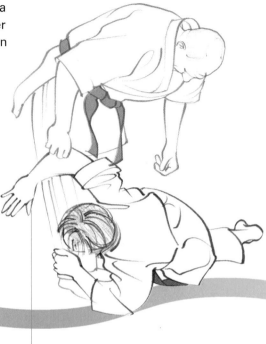

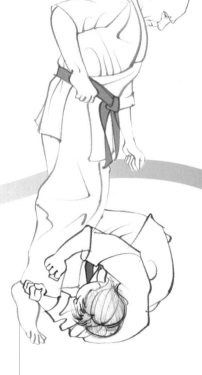

2▲ Having blocked the kick by meeting the attacker's shin with the bony underside of your forearms, 'bridge up' onto your left knee, wrapping your right arm behind the attacker's right knee.

1▲ The attacker attempts a soccer-type kick towards your face and head while you are on the ground in a defensive position, with your forearms protecting your face.

> **TOP TIP**
> Make sure you keep your forearm firmly wedged under the attacker's ankle/lower shin while rolling back against his knee in step 3, to maximize the effect of the lower-leg lock.

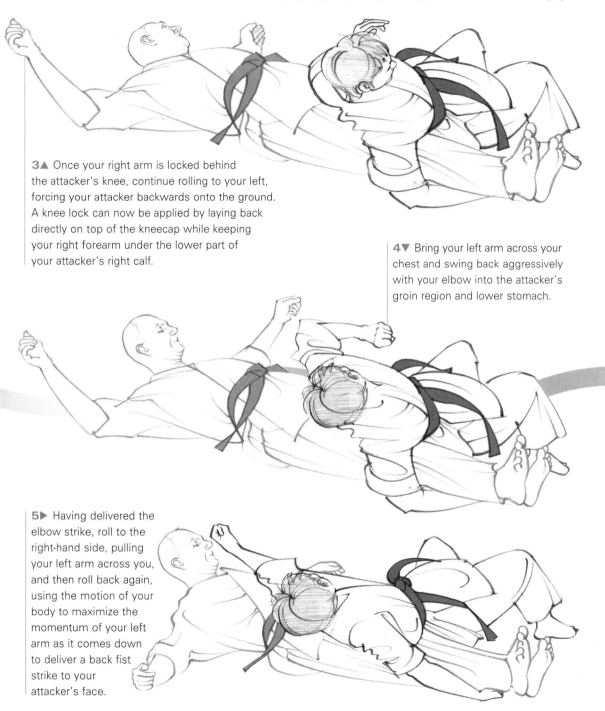

3▲ Once your right arm is locked behind the attacker's knee, continue rolling to your left, forcing your attacker backwards onto the ground. A knee lock can now be applied by laying back directly on top of the kneecap while keeping your right forearm under the lower part of your attacker's right calf.

4▼ Bring your left arm across your chest and swing back aggressively with your elbow into the attacker's groin region and lower stomach.

5► Having delivered the elbow strike, roll to the right-hand side, pulling your left arm across you, and then roll back again, using the motion of your body to maximize the momentum of your left arm as it comes down to deliver a back fist strike to your attacker's face.

Rear strangles from kneeling (1)

This technique is singularly one of the most effective chokes within Ju-Jitsu's vast repertoire, due to the fact that it does not rely on the attacker's clothing to effect the strangle or choke.

2▼ Bring your left arm across and rest it on the top of your attacker's left shoulder, with your palm facing uppermost. Grab your left bicep with your right hand.

1▲ With the attacker sitting on the floor in front of you, kneel down behind him, bringing your right forearm across the front of his throat and under his chin.

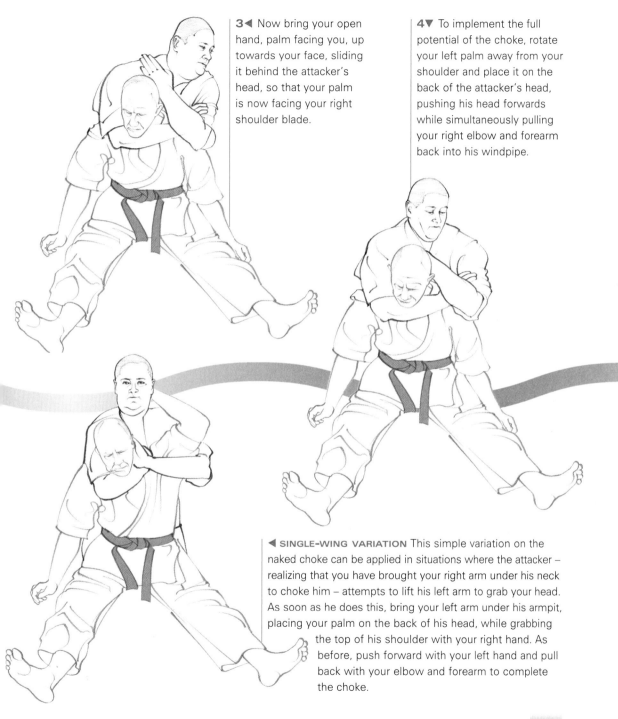

3◄ Now bring your open hand, palm facing you, up towards your face, sliding it behind the attacker's head, so that your palm is now facing your right shoulder blade.

4▼ To implement the full potential of the choke, rotate your left palm away from your shoulder and place it on the back of the attacker's head, pushing his head forwards while simultaneously pulling your right elbow and forearm back into his windpipe.

◄ SINGLE-WING VARIATION This simple variation on the naked choke can be applied in situations where the attacker – realizing that you have brought your right arm under his neck to choke him – attempts to lift his left arm to grab your head. As soon as he does this, bring your left arm under his armpit, placing your palm on the back of his head, while grabbing the top of his shoulder with your right hand. As before, push forward with your left hand and pull back with your elbow and forearm to complete the choke.

Rear strangles from kneeling (2)

The two techniques shown here are very simple, yet effective, strangles that can be applied to an attacker wearing loose clothing.

COLLAR AND ELBOW 2▼ Slide your right elbow across your chest and place the bony tip against the temple of your attacker. Push your elbow into the temple while at the same time pulling his collar in the opposite direction with your left hand.

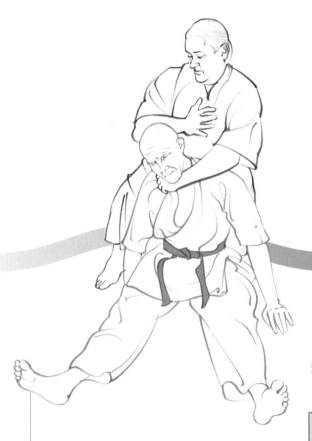

COLLAR AND ELBOW 1▲ Kneeling down on your left knee behind your attacker, bring your left arm under the chin and across the windpipe, grabbing hold of the attacker's collar, while pushing down on the back of his head with your right forearm to prevent any attempt at escaping.

TOP TIP
To maximize the effect of the rather unpleasant technique in the collar-and-elbow method, it's important to get equal leverage on the side of the temple and on the lapel. Resist the temptation to push the head too far over with your elbow, as this will cause your elbow to slide off, thus losing you your advantage.

SLIDING COLLAR AND LAPEL 1▼
Kneel down on your left knee behind your attacker, bringing your right arm under his chin and across the airway, taking a high grip on the back of his collar with your thumb and fingers.

SLIDING COLLAR AND LAPEL 2▼
Now bring your left arm across the attacker's chest and grab halfway down his right lapel, while pulling him firmly into your chest to minimize the risk of escape.

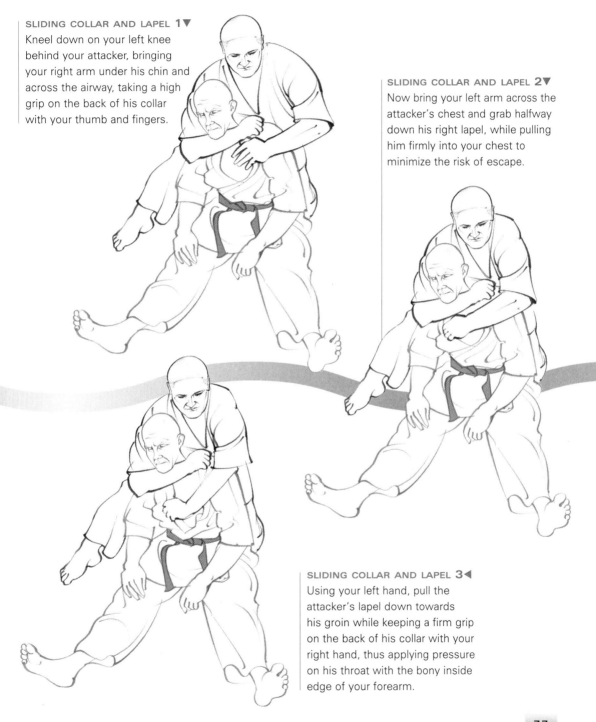

SLIDING COLLAR AND LAPEL 3◄
Using your left hand, pull the attacker's lapel down towards his groin while keeping a firm grip on the back of his collar with your right hand, thus applying pressure on his throat with the bony inside edge of your forearm.

Front strangle from kneeling (1)

This technique relies on the attacker's clothing to effect the strangle, and is known as the 'sleeve wheel', due to the series of movements involved.

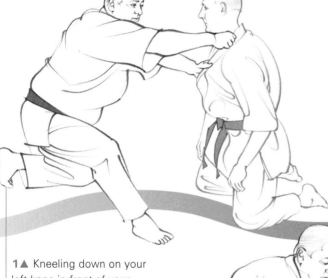

> **TOP TIP**
> This strangle can be used in the standing or kneeling position, or – in some cases – when both parties are prone on the ground. Although requiring a little more practice than some of the other strangles, it has the advantage of often catching your opponent completely unawares.

1▲ Kneeling down on your left knee in front of your attacker, take a high grip on his lapel with your right hand, with your thumb on the inside, while taking a lower grip on the same side with your left hand, but this time with your fingers on the inside.

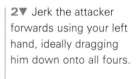

2▼ Jerk the attacker forwards using your left hand, ideally dragging him down onto all fours.

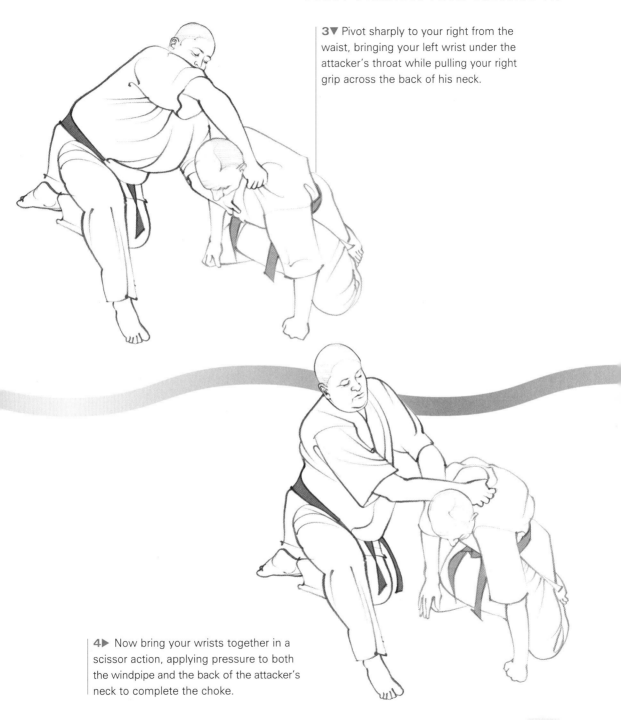

3▼ Pivot sharply to your right from the waist, bringing your left wrist under the attacker's throat while pulling your right grip across the back of his neck.

4▶ Now bring your wrists together in a scissor action, applying pressure to both the windpipe and the back of the attacker's neck to complete the choke.

Front strangle from kneeling (2)

This technique is an excellent move for close-in fighting on the ground, although it can also be applied in a standing scenario equally effectively.

> **TOP TIP**
> To maximize the efficiency of the reclining head throw in step 4, you need to be squatting on the balls of both feet while pulling the attacker's head tightly under your right armpit, maintaining close body contact at all times.

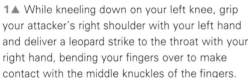

2▼ Having delivered the strike to the throat, immediately pull your right elbow back and initiate a follow-up attack – again to the throat – using your right forearm.

1▲ While kneeling down on your left knee, grip your attacker's right shoulder with your left hand and deliver a leopard strike to the throat with your right hand, bending your fingers over to make contact with the middle knuckles of the fingers.

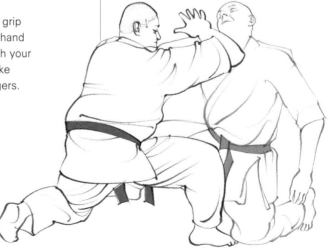

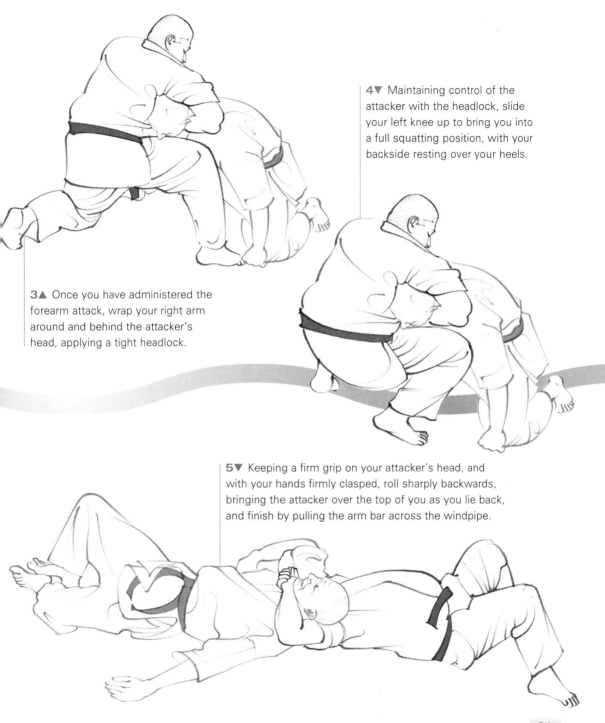

4▼ Maintaining control of the attacker with the headlock, slide your left knee up to bring you into a full squatting position, with your backside resting over your heels.

3▲ Once you have administered the forearm attack, wrap your right arm around and behind the attacker's head, applying a tight headlock.

5▼ Keeping a firm grip on your attacker's head, and with your hands firmly clasped, roll sharply backwards, bringing the attacker over the top of you as you lie back, and finish by pulling the arm bar across the windpipe.

DEFENCE AGAINST EDGED WEAPONS

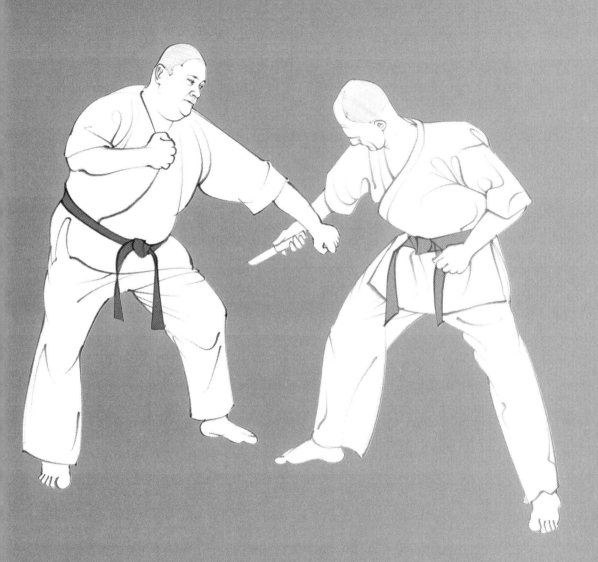

Straight-arm lock against knife

Control is vital when dealing with a knife attack, in order to minimize the risk of injury. Here, the weapon arm is safely secured using a straight-arm-lock counter – in this case against a knife threat to the stomach.

TOP TIP
To maximize the effect of the arm lock, ensure that your left shoulder is pulled back into the attacker and that your shoulders remain in line with one another.

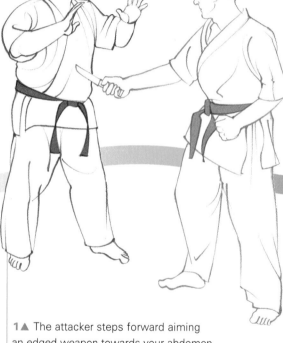

2▼ Turning sharply to your right, and thus rapidly closing the gap between you and the attacker, use your right hand to secure the wrist of the knife-wielding hand, while using your left elbow to strike inside the attacker's elbow joint, bringing him even closer towards you.

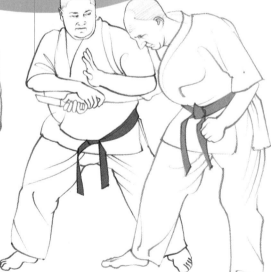

1▲ The attacker steps forward aiming an edged weapon towards your abdomen. Respond by immediately stepping back with your right foot into a passive defensive stance, to communicate that you don't want any trouble.

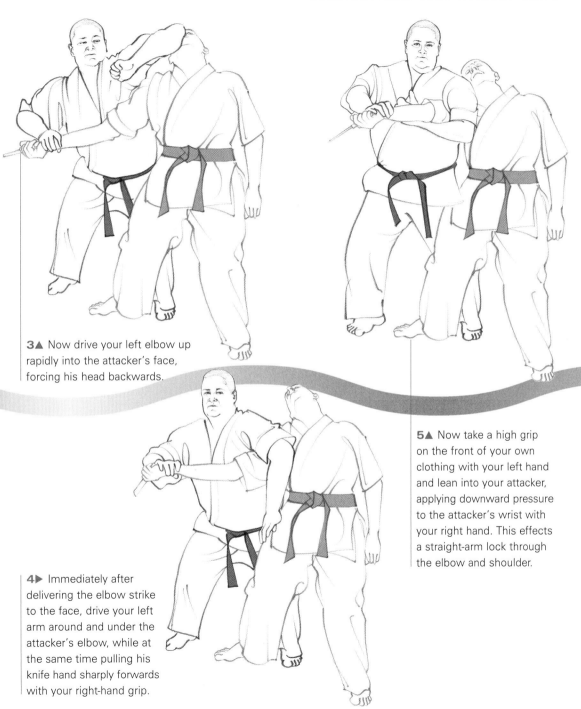

3▲ Now drive your left elbow up rapidly into the attacker's face, forcing his head backwards.

5▲ Now take a high grip on the front of your own clothing with your left hand and lean into your attacker, applying downward pressure to the attacker's wrist with your right hand. This effects a straight-arm lock through the elbow and shoulder.

4▶ Immediately after delivering the elbow strike to the face, drive your left arm around and under the attacker's elbow, while at the same time pulling his knife hand sharply forwards with your right-hand grip.

Knife threat to neck

This sequence demonstrates how to handle an attack with a knife-like weapon to the neck, using a skilled, controlled response to minimize the risk.

1▼ The attacker threatens you by holding an edged weapon to the side of your neck. Step back on your left leg, raising your hands and adopting the passive defensive stance in response to the threat, to indicate that you are 'backing off' from the attack.

2▼ Pivot to the left, using the palm of your right hand to push the attacker's weapon hand away from your neck. Then use the back of your left hand to block the weapon hand and prevent the attacker from slashing with the weapon at close contact.

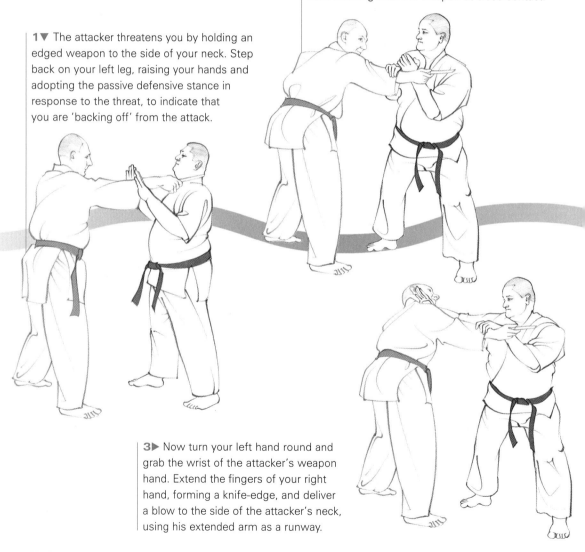

3▶ Now turn your left hand round and grab the wrist of the attacker's weapon hand. Extend the fingers of your right hand, forming a knife-edge, and deliver a blow to the side of the attacker's neck, using his extended arm as a runway.

4▶ Draw your right hand back to your chest and, stepping in closer to the attacker, execute an elbow strike to the side of his head (maximize the impact by pulling the attacker's weapon hand to the left and across your body with your left hand while simultaneously delivering the strike).

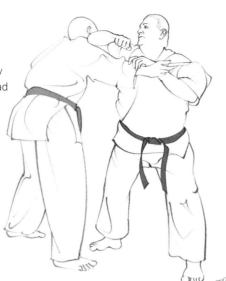

6▼ With a firm grip on the attacker's head, pivot sharply to the right, rotating your hips. At the same time, push the attacker's head downwards while bringing your left knee up to deliver a blow to his jaw.

5▼ Immediately after striking the attacker, raise both your arms and place them on the back of his head in preparation for the finishing strike.

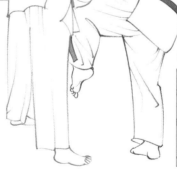

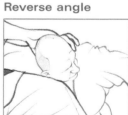

Reverse angle

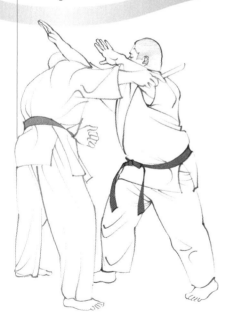

TOP TIP
This technique relies on the principle of action being faster than reaction. Using your right palm to parry the weapon away from your neck allows you to jam your left wrist between the attacker's wrist and your body before he is able to react.

Knife threat to stomach

This technique demonstrates how to respond safely to a lunge with an edged weapon to the stomach, the final blow of the sequence enabling you to secure the weapon from the attacker.

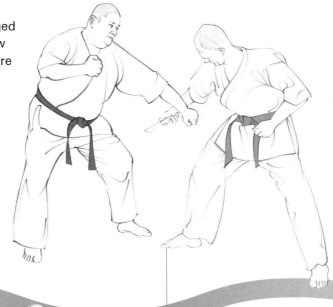

1▼ The attacker readies himself to lunge at you with an edged weapon, so bring yourself into guard stance with your left leg leading, so that you are ready to counter-attack.

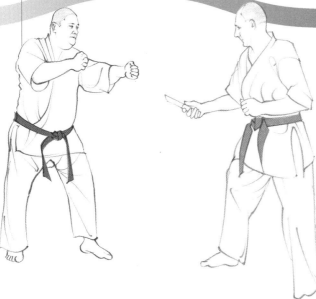

2▲ As the attacker lunges with his knife, sweep your left arm down to parry the blade to the left-hand side of your body.

TOP TIP
To maximize the effect of the final knockout blow to the head using the shin, it is vital to maintain the straightness of the kicking leg throughout the movement.

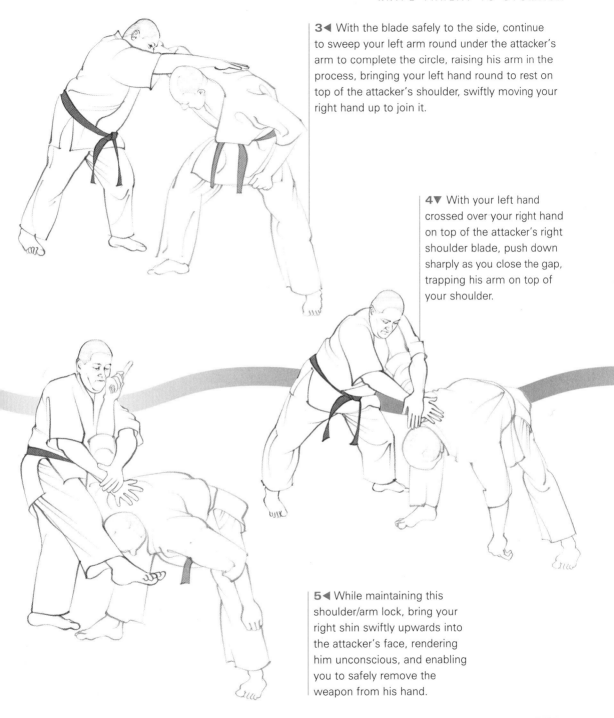

3◄ With the blade safely to the side, continue to sweep your left arm round under the attacker's arm to complete the circle, raising his arm in the process, bringing your left hand round to rest on top of the attacker's shoulder, swiftly moving your right hand up to join it.

4▼ With your left hand crossed over your right hand on top of the attacker's right shoulder blade, push down sharply as you close the gap, trapping his arm on top of your shoulder.

5◄ While maintaining this shoulder/arm lock, bring your right shin swiftly upwards into the attacker's face, rendering him unconscious, and enabling you to safely remove the weapon from his hand.

Knife threat to back

This knife-defence technique demonstrates how to deal with an attack from behind, when an assailant has a knife held to your back.

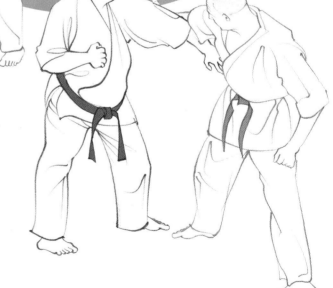

TOP TIP
The speed at which you drop to your left knee, and thus bring your attacker's face crashing down onto your kneecap in a finishing blow, will ultimately dictate the outcome of this sequence.

2▼ Turn swiftly to your left, with your left arm parrying the blade away from you in preparation for your follow-up counter-attack.

1▲ The attacker has moved in behind you, to threaten you from the rear. Maintain a passive defensive stance, with your hands held high enough for your attacker to see, all the while looking over your left shoulder in readiness to respond to the threat.

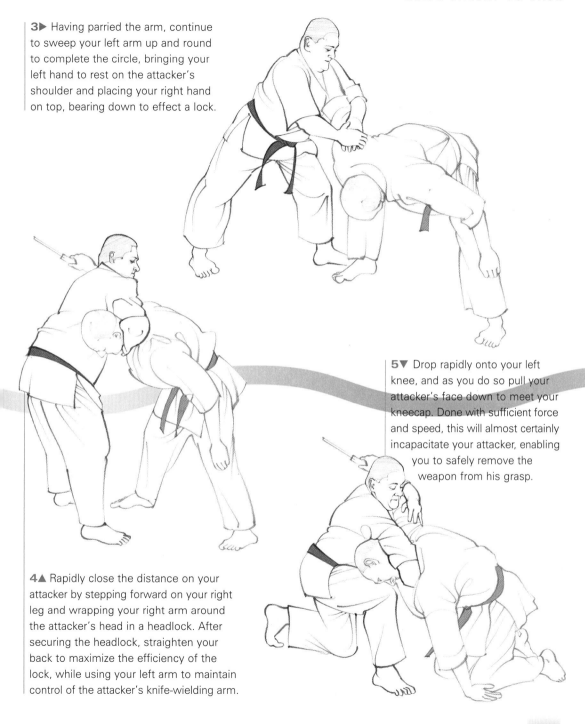

3▶ Having parried the arm, continue to sweep your left arm up and round to complete the circle, bringing your left hand to rest on the attacker's shoulder and placing your right hand on top, bearing down to effect a lock.

5▼ Drop rapidly onto your left knee, and as you do so pull your attacker's face down to meet your kneecap. Done with sufficient force and speed, this will almost certainly incapacitate your attacker, enabling you to safely remove the weapon from his grasp.

4▲ Rapidly close the distance on your attacker by stepping forward on your right leg and wrapping your right arm around the attacker's head in a headlock. After securing the headlock, straighten your back to maximize the efficiency of the lock, while using your left arm to maintain control of the attacker's knife-wielding arm.

Roundhouse bottle attack

It is important to learn the basics of defence against a bottle attack in your Ju-Jitsu training. The sequence shown here can be applied when an attacker swings a bottle round at you from the side, in a roundhouse attack.

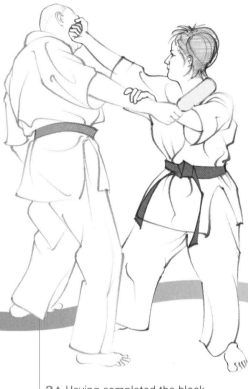

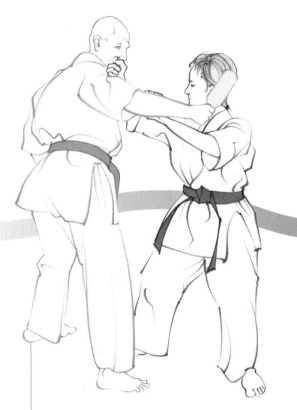

2▲ Having completed the block, use your right fist to counter-strike by delivering a back fist strike to the side of the attacker's face, making contact with your knuckles.

1▲ The attacker swings the bottle round in a circular action towards your head. Block his arm with your left hand, at the same time using your right fist to strike in a downward hammer action to the bicep.

TOP TIP
Remember that, although there is no major strike to complete this sequence, you have removed the bottle or weapon from your attacker, and are now able to use this to your potential advantage.

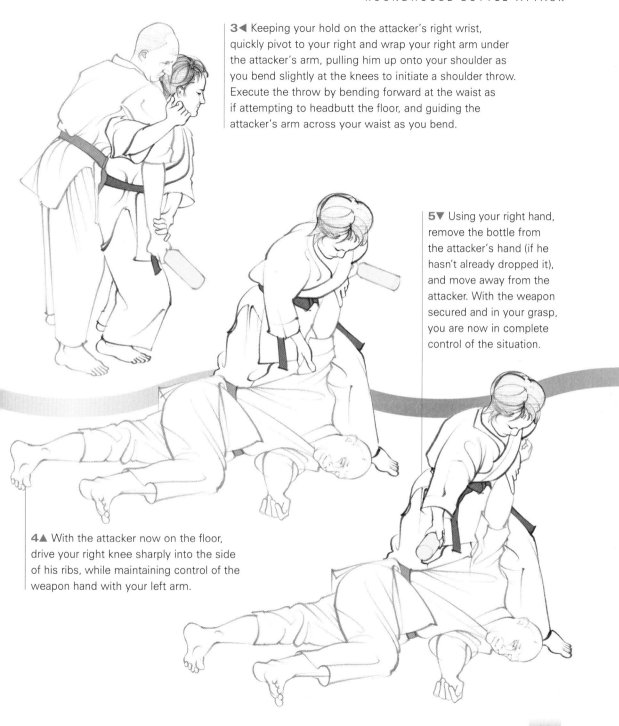

3◀ Keeping your hold on the attacker's right wrist, quickly pivot to your right and wrap your right arm under the attacker's arm, pulling him up onto your shoulder as you bend slightly at the knees to initiate a shoulder throw. Execute the throw by bending forward at the waist as if attempting to headbutt the floor, and guiding the attacker's arm across your waist as you bend.

5▼ Using your right hand, remove the bottle from the attacker's hand (if he hasn't already dropped it), and move away from the attacker. With the weapon secured and in your grasp, you are now in complete control of the situation.

4▲ With the attacker now on the floor, drive your right knee sharply into the side of his ribs, while maintaining control of the weapon hand with your left arm.

Slashing bottle attack

This technique shows how to defend against a roundhouse slashing action with a bottle aimed towards the side of the head and face.

1▼ The attacker raises the bottle above his head in an attempt to slash across your face. Step back straight away into the guard stance, to ready yourself for your counter-attack.

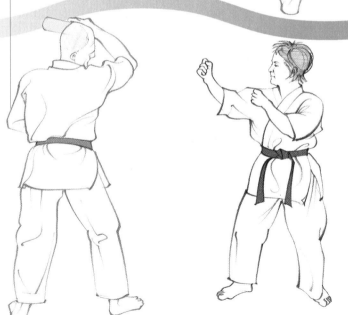

2▲ As the attacking arm swings round towards you, step outwards onto your left foot and parry the attacking hand with your right forearm. Having blocked the attack, immediately counter with a follow-up palm-heel strike across the attacker's jaw, using your left hand, taking a grip on his right wrist with your right hand.

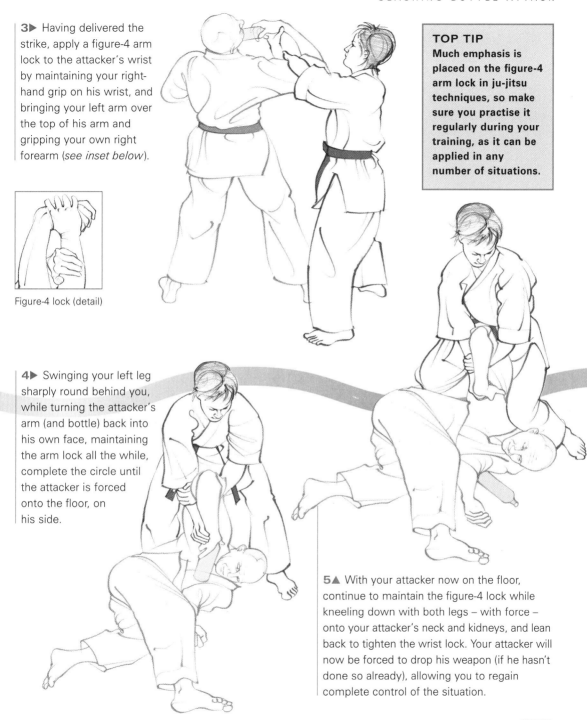

3▶ Having delivered the strike, apply a figure-4 arm lock to the attacker's wrist by maintaining your right-hand grip on his wrist, and bringing your left arm over the top of his arm and gripping your own right forearm (*see inset below*).

Figure-4 lock (detail)

TOP TIP
Much emphasis is placed on the figure-4 arm lock in ju-jitsu techniques, so make sure you practise it regularly during your training, as it can be applied in any number of situations.

4▶ Swinging your left leg sharply round behind you, while turning the attacker's arm (and bottle) back into his own face, maintaining the arm lock all the while, complete the circle until the attacker is forced onto the floor, on his side.

5▲ With your attacker now on the floor, continue to maintain the figure-4 lock while kneeling down with both legs – with force – onto your attacker's neck and kidneys, and lean back to tighten the wrist lock. Your attacker will now be forced to drop his weapon (if he hasn't done so already), allowing you to regain complete control of the situation.

Overhead bottle attack (1)

This defence sequence shows how to deal with an attacker who is threatening you with an overhead bottle strike. As always, a controlled response is vital in order to minimize the risk of injury from the weapon.

2▼ As the bottle drops towards your head, step into the attack using a rising front block with the bony outer edge of your left forearm, to prevent the bottle from reaching its target.

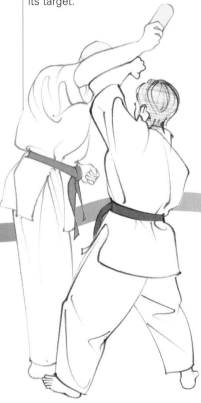

1▲ The attacker raises the bottle above his head in an attempt to strike you. Step quickly into your guard stance, left leg leading, in preparation for your counter-move.

TOP TIP
The hip twist in step 3 generates momentum and increases the power of your elbow strike. Without this added power, your strike may not have the desired effect on your attacker.

3▼ Having blocked the attack, twist your hips to the left, while simultaneously delivering an elbow strike to the attacker's floating ribs with your right arm.

4▼ After executing the elbow strike, bring your right hand up and over the top of the attacker's wrist, placing your left hand on top of your right, and pushing the attacker's arm back on itself. Then step out to the side with your left leg.

5▶ Keeping your hold on the attacker's wrist, pivot sharply round to the left, which will unbalance the attacker and drag him to the floor. Once he is down, place your right knee into the top of his shoulder blade, using your body weight to apply pressure, and remove the bottle from his grasp with your right hand.

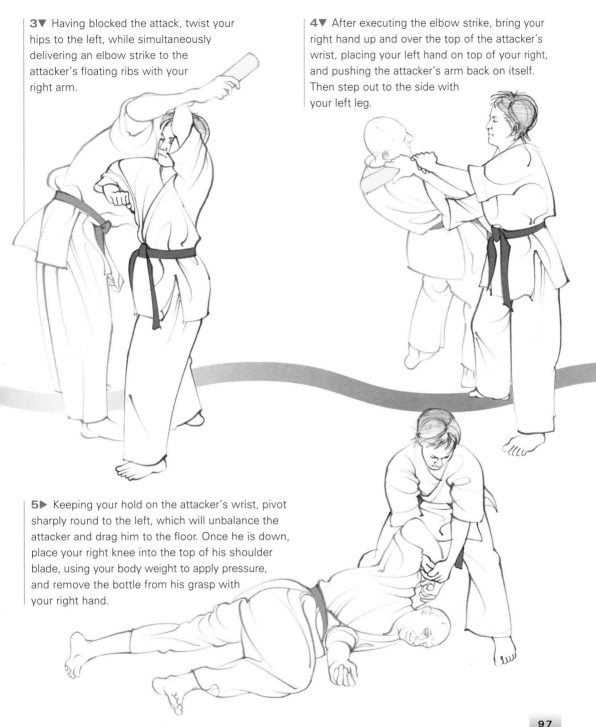

Overhead bottle attack (2)

This technique is a variation of a defence against an overhead strike with a bottle, and is particularly suited to people of a smaller build, due to the mechanics involved.

2▼ As the attacker brings the bottle down towards your head, step in to intercept the attack with a rising front block, using the bony underside of your left forearm.

1▲ The attacker raises the bottle above his head in an attempt to strike you. Immediately step into your guard stance, left leg leading, to ready yourself for the attack.

TOP TIP
To maximize your ability to tip the attacker backwards, ensure that you lift his right upper leg at the same time as driving his face backwards with the palm-heel strike to the nose.

3▼ Having blocked the weapon arm, push your left hand up under the attacker's nose in a palm-heel strike, to drive the attacker's head and shoulders backwards and ultimately throw him off balance. At the same time, bring your right arm up sharply between the attacker's legs to strike the groin.

4▼ Immediately after executing the groin strike with your right arm, bend your arm round the back of the attacker's right leg, and lift the leg as you continue to drive his face backwards with your left hand, toppling the attacker to the ground.

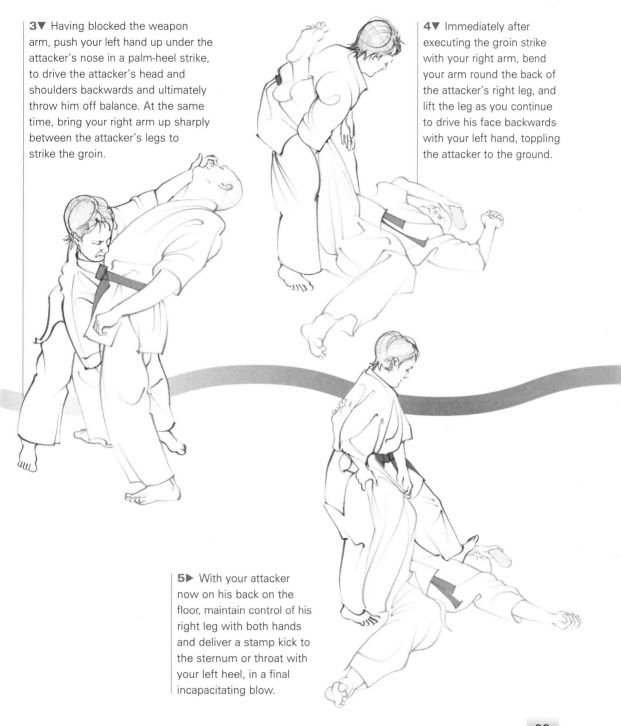

5▶ With your attacker now on his back on the floor, maintain control of his right leg with both hands and deliver a stamp kick to the sternum or throat with your left heel, in a final incapacitating blow.

DEFENCE AGAINST ARMED WEAPONS

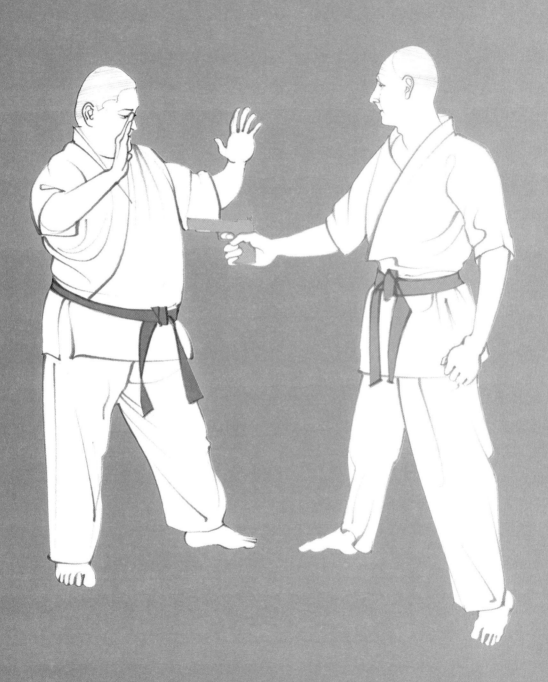

Gun threat to chest (1)

Here we address the increasing problem of a threat with a firearm. Dealing with firearms at close range should only be attempted if there is a serious risk to life, and a high degree of control must be employed at all times while dealing with the threat.

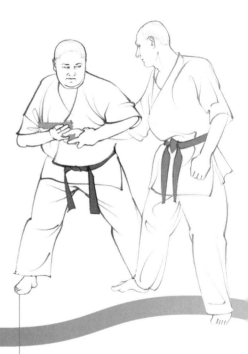

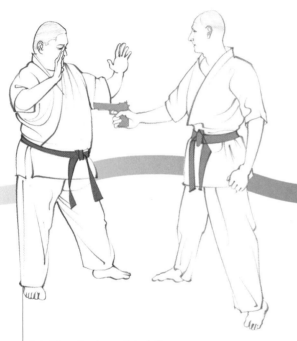

2▲ Pivot rapidly to your right, with your left hand coming over the top of the attacker's weapon arm and securing his hand and the pistol grip to the side of your chest, bringing your right hand up in readiness for the next move.

1▲ The attacker points a firearm directly at your chest, so immediately step back into a passive defensive stance, and don't make any sudden moves until such time as you deem it absolutely necessary.

> **TOP TIP**
> The success of this defence relies solely on the speed at which you pivot in step 2, and move the barrel away from your chest. Remember: action is faster than reaction.

3▼ Bringing your right hand underneath the weapon and gripping your fingers over the top of the pistol, snatch the weapon backwards so that the barrel ends up facing the attacker. This will almost certainly break his trigger finger, which will be caught inside the trigger guard (*see inset below*).

4▼ Snatching the weapon from the attacker's hand, advance on your attacker to close the gap, and strike a devastating blow to his head using the butt of the pistol.

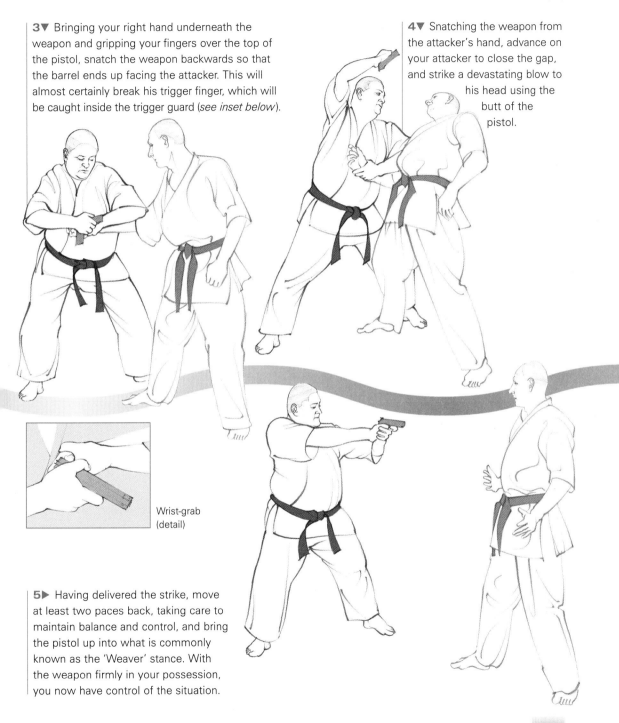

Wrist-grab (detail)

5▶ Having delivered the strike, move at least two paces back, taking care to maintain balance and control, and bring the pistol up into what is commonly known as the 'Weaver' stance. With the weapon firmly in your possession, you now have control of the situation.

Gun threat to chest (2)

This gun-defence technique not only disarms the attacker, but also puts the experienced handler of firearms into a position where he or she can detain and arrest the attacker using the attacker's own weapon.

3▼ Having used both hands to gain control of the wrist holding the firearm, pivot rapidly to your left, bringing the barrel of the firearm round to cover the attacker's chest.

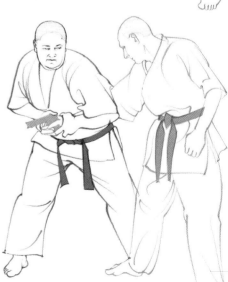

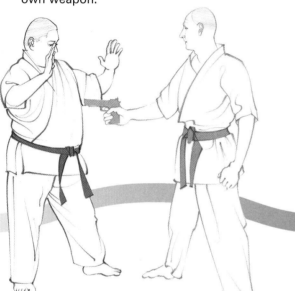

1▲ The attacker points a pistol at your chest, so immediately step back into the passive defensive stance and await your opportunity, keeping your eyes trained on the weapon.

2▶ Twisting sharply to the right, bring your left arm over the top of the attacker's forearm, pointing the barrel away from you and towards the ground, to minimize the risk of anyone else in the vicinity getting caught should the weapon discharge.

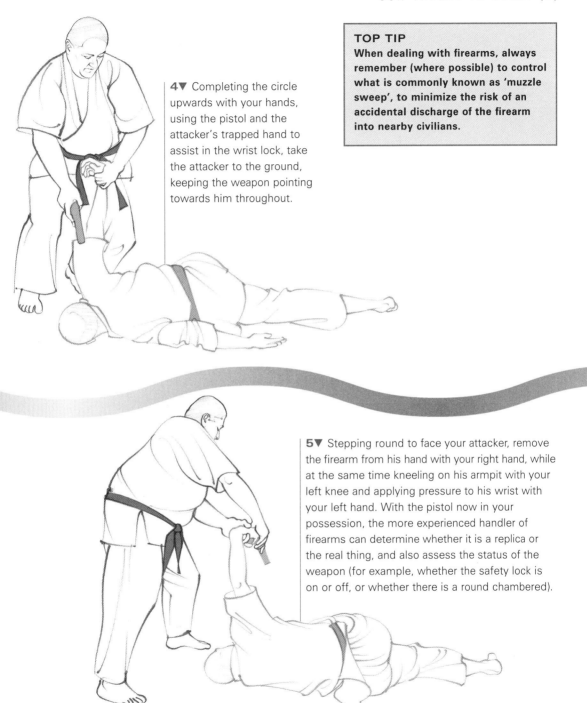

4▼ Completing the circle upwards with your hands, using the pistol and the attacker's trapped hand to assist in the wrist lock, take the attacker to the ground, keeping the weapon pointing towards him throughout.

TOP TIP
When dealing with firearms, always remember (where possible) to control what is commonly known as 'muzzle sweep', to minimize the risk of an accidental discharge of the firearm into nearby civilians.

5▼ Stepping round to face your attacker, remove the firearm from his hand with your right hand, while at the same time kneeling on his armpit with your left knee and applying pressure to his wrist with your left hand. With the pistol now in your possession, the more experienced handler of firearms can determine whether it is a replica or the real thing, and also assess the status of the weapon (for example, whether the safety lock is on or off, or whether there is a round chambered).

Training diary

Index of techniques

Please note:
Full demonstrations of the techniques are shown in **bold**.

About the author

Kevin Pell Hanshi MGRY, 8th Dan black belt, is the founder of Ishin Ryu Ju-Jitsu – a worldwide organization with over 11,000 students. A full-time international instructor, Kevin has been featured on the cover of both *Combat* and *Martial Arts Plus* magazines, and was inaugurated into the prestigious Combat Black Belt Hall of Fame in 2003.

Kevin began martial arts training at age 8 and has, over the last 40 years to date, studied a wide range of arts, including Shorinji-Kempo (which included training at the famous Honbu Dojo in Japan), Judo, Kung Fu, Kickboxing, Iaido and Karate. In his extensive military career, Kevin has served with the Royal Marine Reserve and the Royal Military Police, and served as a dog handler in the parks police. In 1996 he was personally invited to join an elite Close Protection Team drawn from Britain's Special Forces, responsible for the personal security of heads of state within the United Arab Emirates. Kevin also runs SAS Survival School and close-protection training courses, and is a specialist in tactical and defensive knife training.

His custom-built dojo and headquarters in Caston, Norfolk, is fast becoming recognized as an international centre of excellence for the practice of Ju-Jitsu. He is one of the few senior coaches in Great Britain to be officially recognized as a first-generation founder. Visit the Ishin Ryu Ju-Jitsu website at www.ishinryu.com

Acknowledgments

I would like to thank the following for their inspiration, support, guidance and belief in me: the staff at Eddison Sadd Editions, especially Ian, Elaine and Malcolm, and a special thank you to Tessa Monina for her patience and willingness to drive to my home in Norfolk to help me meet the deadline. To all at Rupert Crew Ltd, especially my long-suffering literary agent, Doreen Montgomery.

Special thanks also go to my students Martin Adil-Smith and Stephen Ankier for their invaluable assistance in selecting the techniques and writing them up, and to Sheila Eglen, Martin Bates, Marek Marcek, Thomas Hassey, Emily Bates, and Samantha and Charlotte Taverner for giving up their time to model for the illustrations.

EDDISON•SADD EDITIONS

Editorial Director Ian Jackson
Managing Editor Tessa Monina
Senior Editor Katie Golsby
Art Director Elaine Partington
Mac Designer Brazzle Atkins
Illustrator Juliet Percival
Production Cara Herron

Eddison Sadd would like to thank all those who kindly took part in the reference photography.